# THE LITTLE BIBLE OF 77 CENSORED CURES

# THE LITTLE BIBLE OF 77 CENSORED CURES

*by Laissez Faire Contributors*

Laissez Faire Books

ISBN: 978-1-6212911-9-0 (print)

18 17 16 15 14 1 2 3 4 5 6 7

Published by Laissez Faire Books, 808 St. Paul Street, Baltimore, Maryland
www.lfb.org

Cover and Layout Design: Mena Fusco

# CONTENTS

# INTRODUCTION

If you're going to depend on the Food and Drug Administration to keep you healthy, you're not going to last long. Sure, they'll tell you their mission is to make sure the food and drugs you put in your body are safe. But they've created regulatory burdens that hinder, rather than promote, medical and health innovations. In fact, their system of approving any medical drugs or devices has caused prices to skyrocket and limited what kinds of drugs are researched.

It's a perfect example of the government thinking it's doing the right thing, and screwing everything up in the process.

That's why we've put together this book. We know the government is too busy following the red tape it created to actually care about what's happening to you. So we've scoured the Internet and any medical and health books we could get our hands on to come up with the best natural health solutions you've probably never heard of.

You probably won't hear anyone from the government endorsing these ideas. They haven't gone through the FDA's approval process, which usually takes over ten years to complete. But that doesn't mean you shouldn't trust these health solutions. They've undergone numerous scientific studies.

And more important, many of them have withstood the test of time. They're the same remedies used by people hundreds or thousands of years ago.

In the following pages, you'll find a number of solutions we think will make your life a little better. Maybe you've been having back pain for months and you and your doctor have run out of possible solutions.

Or your sex drive isn't what it once was and you want a natural way to improve it. Maybe you know a friend suffering from cancer and you want to help relieve her pain with a natural remedy.

When we started this project, our goal was to bring you 77 cures that could make your life better. Little did we know we'd come across close to 100 natural health solutions. You could say it was a pleasant surprise.

Check out what we've uncovered for you.

# CHAPTER 1: CANCER CURES

Every year, nearly 2 million Americans are diagnosed with cancer. One person out of every three will receive a cancer diagnosis at some time in their lives — despite 21st century technology advances.

That's a surprising statement. But Western medicine's track record with cancer doesn't look so hot. Consider this:

- In the early 1900s, one in 20 people developed cancer.
- In the 1940s, one in 16 people developed cancer.
- In the 1970s, it was one in 10.
- Today, it's one in three!

How can anybody call this progress… it's beyond me.

Here's the kicker:

For decades, millions of dollars have been funneled into cancer research, yet here we are, with no official cure. It's easy to see why, when you follow the money.

According to the CDC, about 1,660,290 (1.66 million) new cancer cases are expected to be diagnosed in 2013. If overall death rates are falling, why are new diagnosis of cancer on the rise?

The answer is simple: The so-called 40-year "war on cancer" is a scam. The cancer epidemic has been a boon for the bank accounts of big pharma.

The typical cancer patient spends a whopping $50,000 fighting for his life. Chemotherapy drugs are among the most expensive of all medical treatments, with some of them ranging from $3,000 to $7,000 for just a one-month supply.

When it comes to fighting cancer, it's been beaten into our heads that you need chemotherapy drugs, radiotherapy, diagnostic procedures, and surgeries. For most people, this is a frightening ordeal — just from the treatments alone which often cause awful side effects like nausea and loss of hair.

In spite of the enormous amounts of money socked into cancer research, two out of three cancer patients will be dead within five years after receiving cancer surgery, radiotherapy and/or chemotherapy. That's a lousy batting ratio if you ask me.

Here's another shocker most people don't know. A recent study estimated that chemotherapy benefits about one of every 20 people receiving it. And they call this modern day medicine? It sounds like stone-age medicine to me.

And yet — Mother Nature has natural cancer cures available that almost always benefit the overall health of the body. But there's one tiny problem.

All have been vehemently discounted, silenced, and pushed under the rug by the medical monopoly… who routinely persecutes physicians and researchers. The Feds come down on these good Samaritans like common criminals.

Take for instance Greg Caton, who was manufacturing anti-cancer salves that eliminated skin cancer tumors. The Feds planned to shut him down. So Greg left the country for Ecuador which by the way appreciates people who come up with cures. There, Greg could legally help the community with his treatment. However this didn't last long. The Feds found him in Ecuador, kidnapped him, and threw the book at him.

They don't want you to have other options to treat your own body. But we do.

## THE VIRGIN MARY CANCER CURE

Officially, it's a fermented wheat germ extract. But we like to use the name it was originally given by its creator, Dr. Mate Hidvegi. In honor of the Virgin Mary, he named it after the "Hail, Mary." Ave Maria.

He called it **Avemar**.

Before you can understand how this miracle drug works, it's important to understand how cancer works. Then you'll see why Avemar is so effective. Malignant cells that form tumors in the body use higher levels of glucose in order to grow. Because of this, pharmaceutical companies have focused on ways of inhibiting the cancer's ability to metabolize glucose. They believe if they can prevent these cells from breaking down nutrients, they can limit the growth of potentially fatal tumors.

Conventional cancer treatments like chemotherapy and radiation attempts to kill these cancerous cells before they spread and destroy the body. The problem with that, however, is that the treatment can't usually tell the difference between healthy and cancer cells.

That's where Avemar comes in.

Dr. Hidvegi's discovery targets the glucose metabolism of cancer cells. By preventing these cells from breaking down glucose, it prevents them from creating the building blocks of additional cancer cells, stimulating cell death in tumors. There have even been reports that Avemar helped increase weight gain in cancer patients, and made their bodies even more tolerant of traditional cancer treatments. Cancer patients who routinely use the product feel more energetic, experience less pain, and have an improved quality of life.

But that's not the only thing Avemar can do. It also assists your body's immune system in identifying and destroying foreign or abnormal cells in the body. Avemar suppresses a cancer cell's ability to release a masking agent that normally hides it from your body's white blood cells. Additionally, it's been shown to restore the body's bone marrow ability to create new red blood cells.

Avemar is non-toxic, but don't take it if you're currently pregnant or breastfeeding, or if you've had an organ transplant.

## THE "ALLIGATOR PEAR" THAT CAN SHRINK TUMORS

Avocados provide the body with many health benefits due to the high number of vitamins and minerals found within. How? They contain powerful antioxidants that help reverse the effects of many illnesses.

Contained within each avocado are plant chemicals known as "phytochemicals." This substance protects the body by reducing the risk of major chronic illnesses such as cancer. Phytochemicals in avocados also include lutein, glutathione and oleic acid. Lutein reduces breast cancer, while glutathione, an antioxidant, allows the liver to detoxify the body quickly and even reduce the effects of stress. Oleic acid, a healthy monounsaturated fat, lowers LDL cholesterol. This promotes a healthy heart, and helps prevent other harmful health side effects.

Vitamin E is also an important antioxidant for cancer prevention. When vitamin E is digested directly from a food source, it creates cancer-protective layers within the body that reduce the chances of developing cancer. However, vitamin E from synthetic sources (such as alpha tocopherol acetate), do not possess cancer preventive layers. Avocados are a true vitamin E source.

Known as "the Alligator Pear" in the south, this fruit reduces the risk of cancer when consumed with other healthy meals.

---

**Did you know that taking vitamin E along with vitamin C can also reduce your chances of having a heart attack. These vitamins help expand and dilate your arteries and blood vessels, decreasing the chance of a major heart attack. In fact, take them before a fatty meal to decrease your chances of something bad happening.**

---

## THE SKIN CANCER SAVIORS

**Fava beans** contain low amounts of saturated fat and cholesterol. But they're still loaded with vitamins and minerals you need to live a healthy lifestyle. Eating fava beans provides you with high concentrations of potassium, vitamin K, vitamin B-6, magnesium, zinc, selenium and thiamin. It can also help prevent potential health ailments like neurological diseases, heart disease and cancers.

After the beans have been blanched and shelled, fava beans give you a ton of vitamins and minerals. In fact, one cup of fava beans contains roughly 177 mg of folate, 44% of the recommend daily value for both men and women. Consumption of folate can help improve the nervous system, as well as the production of RNA, DNA, and even red blood cells. Foliate also creates a protective barrier in the blood stream and around organs, reducing the risk of cancer significantly.

The beans also contain a high level of fiber, supplying 37% of your daily recommended dietary value. A high fiber diet can reduce the chances of cancer by ensuring consistent bowel movements.

Likewise, soy **isoflavinoids** create a similar effect as fava beans because of its high fiber content. It goes a step further, however. Soy isoflavinoids lower the risk of breast, uterine, and prostate cancer by creating phytoestrogens, which promotes anti-estrogenic behavior.

## THE NATURAL INDIAN CANCER SECRET

Curry powder is another "super food" because it contains the substance **turmeric**. This antioxidant powder packs a powerful punch acting as both an anti-inflammatory as well as having anticancer properties.

"Curcumin" is a compound located inside of the turmeric spice. Studies have shown this compound helps reduce inflammation in the body. It's so powerful, in fact, it can help reduce pain and inflammation associated with osteoarthritis and rheumatoid arthritis.

However, its anticancer properties are what's most interesting about it. After several preliminary studies, curcumin has been shown to prevent colorectal cancers from forming. The compound seems to stabilize any malignant cells, stopping them from progressing any further. This then allows the patient to recover on their own.

Studies are still being conducted to confirm these findings. Regardless, there is a strong link between eating healthy portions of turmeric and reducing your risk of developing certain cancers.

## A CANCER CURE HIDDEN IN YOUR SPICE RACK

You most likely have this next natural cure in your pantry. We're talking about **black pepper**. This household condiment does more than season food. There've been documented cases of pepper strengthening a person's health and warding off diseases.

Recent cell research has shown that pepper also has anti-inflammatory, antioxidant, and anticancer properties. What makes this compound so powerful? The compound prevents certain cancers (like stomach and colon cancer) from forming within your body. The more pepper you eat, the better your chances of fending off certain ailments and improving your overall health.

When eating black pepper, it's best to combine it with curcumin to increase the impact of both substances. In other words, you can enhance the anticancer and anti-inflammatory properties by eating them together. Eating it alongside epigallocatechin gallate (a substance commonly found in green tea) also boosts its potency.

**Since we're talking about green tea, here are some important things to know about the powerful substance. When buying the product, make sure you buy the freshest tea available, i.e. the ones with the latest expiration date. And remember to get the ones served in individual packs. That's the best way to preserve the tea's powerful natural healing effects. And finally, avoid green tea if you're pregnant or trying to become pregnant. Green tea is a angiogenesis inhibitor, which means it inhibits the growth of new blood vessels.**

## THE CANCER CURE YOUR KIDS ALREADY LOVE

Red and green **grapes** are more than a sweet treat you feed your kids. This super fruit, including its leaves and sap, are used as a remedy for many diseases due to its high antioxidant power.

Grapes assist with cardiovascular ailments such as poor circulation and high cholesterol. You can even alleviate some symptoms associated with diabetes. Make sure you eat both the skin and the seeds to help prevent certain cancers from even forming. The fruit also has an antioxidant that inhibits the growth of malignant cells and may even cause a retrogression in certain cancers.

Many tests done on grapes, however, are still in the "preliminary lab" stages. Additional research is still taking place to determine why they help reduce cancers. Regardless, the proven cardiovascular benefits and potential anticancer properties should be enough of a reason to keep eating them.

**Another easy way to get your daily fill of antioxidants is to take Natura Nectar's Red Bee Propolis. It's a natural byproduct of honey production by bees, and it contains 300% more antioxidants than acai!**

## FORTIFY YOUR PROSTATE WITH THIS COMMON VITAMIN

**Vitamin C** provides your body with an essential nutrient necessary for it to function. However, the body doesn't naturally produce this water-soluble vitamin. It's up to you to obtain the vitamin from outside sources. But don't worry, there are plenty of foods available that contain the essential nutrient.

Vitamin C improves your skin's complexion, blood circulation, strengthen ligaments, cartilage, and tendons and even promotes bone health. It will also reduce fevers, and shorten colds if you're unlucky enough to catch one.

Scientific studies on Vitamin C have shown that, if consumed via fruits and vegetables, it can help reduce the risk of developing certain types of cancer. These include: cervix, stomach, pancreas, esophagus, larynx, rectal, breast, lung and colon. Studies have shown that people with high vitamin C diets have a 50% lower risk of getting cancer than those with low vitamin C diets.

---

**While we're on the topic of prostate cancer, here's another simple way to decrease your chances of getting it. Eat more fat. Seriously. Conjugated linoleic acid (CLA) is formed after a change in the structural form of linoleic acid, a common unsaturated fat found in many foods. Studies have shown high levels of CLA reduce the incident rate of breast cancer by up to 50%. Spending a couple of minutes a day making yourself a sandwich with meats high in CLA could save you the agony of having a swollen prostate in the future.**

---

## THE BUTCHER SHOP CANCER SECRET

An unlikely food source in cancer prevention and inhibition is **beef liver**. Eat enough of it and it can actually reduce the number of free radicals in your body. These are harmful substances that form as a result of various chemical processes that occur in your body's different biological systems.

One slice of liver contains more than 420% of your daily-recommended value of vitamin A. This substance is a powerful antioxidant that lines the body with a protective layer and lowers the risk of certain cancers. It can also destroy any free radicals present in the body, helping you fend off potentially dangerous diseases. Since cancers are often caused by free radicals, eliminating them prevents problems from developing later on.

This type of meat is also high in riboflavin and vitamin B12. Combined with vitamin A, they eradicate free radicals and inhibit the growth of certain cancers. Just one or two servings a week can lower your cancer risk by as much as 50%.

**Speaking of vitamin A, did you know one recent study showed that taking up to 1,200 micrograms could reduce your risk of developing melanoma, a type of skin cancer.**

## HOW A VIRGIN SCREWDRIVER COULD PROTECT YOU AGAINST CANCER

Recent scientific studies have shown that **oranges** play a significant role in reducing cancer development.Vitamin C, a major vitamin inside oranges and other citrus foods, is a powerful anticancer food. However, oranges offer more than just Vitamin C.

The pulp of the orange, also known as "orange oil," contains a powerful phytonutrient known as limonene. Oranges and other citrus fruits such as mandarins, lemons and limes all have high levels of this phytonutrient.

Limonene stimulates the body's antioxidant detoxification system, preventing cancers from forming. Additionally, the phytonutrient reduces the activity of a particular protein that could cause an excessive growth of cells, reducing the chance of developing benign cancers. Eating oranges can help reduce cancer by up to 50% and should be a regular staple food in your diet.

**Ask your doctor about intravenous vitamin C infusion. High dosages of vitamin C administered in this fashion improved the quality of life and well-being of cancer patients.**

## THE ALL NATURAL POST-MENOPAUSAL CURE

**Vitamin B** (in all its forms) provides a necessary balance of essential nutrients that help promote growth, development and other health functions in your body.

The various forms of vitamin B are: Thiamin (B1), riboflavin (B2), niacin (B3), pantothenic acid (B5), pyridoxine (B6), biotin (B7), folic acid/folate (B9) and cobalamin (B12). These vitamins fall under the "Vitamin C" category and help play a major role in enzyme activities, protein regulation, and turning food to energy.

Even after a series of randomized tests, no one fully understands why vitamin B reduces your chance of developing cancer. People with higher vitamin B levels have a better chance of living healthier, happier lives and have less of a chance of developing cancer in the future.

---

**Consider taking a multivitamin to cover as many bases as possible. You can get all the nutrients you need in one tab, making it easy to remember and stay on schedule. On top of that, simply taking a multivitamin could reduce your chance of getting cancer by up to 12%!**

---

## POPEYE'S SECRET INGREDIENT

Maybe Popeye was onto something. The colorful cartoon you might have watched on TV when you were younger helped get millions of kids to eat their **spinach**. One can of the green plant would provide him with superhuman strength, giving him an edge over his rival Bluto, and allowing him to save Olive Oyl.

Spinach might not give you muscles like they did on the show, but it still has plenty of nutritional benefits. Enough to make it a part of your everyday diet.

A recent study in Japan showed that glyconutrients, a substance found in spinach, inhibit cancer cell growth and tumor cell growth. The study also showed the nutrients were able to prevent the destruction of DNA in the body. Mice with colon cancer experienced a 56% decrease in tumor size in just two weeks.

Spinach can help prevent from multiple forms of cancer, such as colon, ovarian, and prostate cancer. The more you eat, the better your body will absorb these important nutrients.

## AN ASIAN DELICACY WITH CANCER KILLING PROPERTIES

**Mushrooms** are one of the few edible fungus we know of. Some people might think they're "unpleasant" to eat because it's a fungus. But they couldn't be further from the truth. If you eat the right ones, such as Shiitake, this "super food" could provide you with a wealth of essential nutrients. Mushrooms provide you with the stuff that fights the progression of cancer and AIDS by aiding the body's immune system. In a clinical trial, shiitake mushrooms were able to reduce the harmful symptoms of a person diagnosed with advanced stomach and colorectal cancer.

Cancer-fighting substances are prevalent throughout the fungus. In its purest form, these same substances can be administered to current cancer patients to treat certain stomach and colorectal cancer.

Adding mushrooms to your daily diet, along with a healthy serving of fruits and vegetables can significantly decrease your chances of developing some cancers and help you live a longer, happier life.

## YOUR LAST STAND DEFENSE AGAINST CANCER

Sutherlandia frutescens or "**cancer bush**" is an herb grown in South Africa and Botswana. When fully matured, these bushes reach up to one foot with distinct leaves and deep-red attractive flowers. Though valued by many or ornamental reasons, this plant is also used by locals as a potent cure-all immune system booster.

There have also been claims that it can fight AIDS, cancer, diabetes and other diseases. This has drawn the attention of scientists looking to understand its healing properties. One study showed the "cancer bush" was able to inhibit the growth of specific cancer cells by as much as 50%. Another study confirmed the plant's extract can kill carcinoma cells.

## THE BABY BACK RIBS CANCER CURE ALL

Formally known as "nigella sativa," **black cumin** has gained recent acclaim for being another potential anticancer food. Though this praise is relatively new, many people in eastern cultures have been taking advantage of its amazing healing properties for centuries.

Regardless, black cumin is a food filled with anticancer properties. A study in 1997 by the Cancer Research Laboratory showed black cumin was able to reduce tumor growth by 50%. Additionally it helped increase the growth of bone marrow by over 250%. Additional studies of the "miracle plant" showed that it helped prevent and inhibit the growth of the following cancers: pancreatic, colon, breast, cervical, brain, leukemia, oral and even liver.

The food possesses enzymes that protect the outer layers of all organs. The plant is not only able to inhibit the growth of cancer cells, but it could also reduce the size of the cancer and all but eliminate it.

## THE FRAT BOY CANCER DIET

When you think of a tomato, the first thing that might come to your mind is its color. The red pigment is a color unlike many others. Did you know you could find the same pigment in peppers? And did you know this pigment could potentially save your life.

Known as "**lycopene**," it's a powerful antioxidant with anticancer properties. Lycopene-rich diets (tomatoes only) were shown to result in lower instances of prostate cancer. Other promising results were shown with brain, cervix, breast, mouth, pancreas and even colon and rectum cancer.

Although studies still are ongoing to prove the validity of lycopene's effect on cancer cells, if you're a man, it might be a good idea to increase the number of tomatoes you eat. Just in case…

---

**Fun fact, did you know that red peppers actually have more vitamin C than oranges. Remember that the next time you go shopping and want a vitamin C alternative.**

---

## A CANCER REMEDY AND A WEIGHT LOSS SOLUTION ALL IN ONE

Up until the 1930s, Americans were losing the cancer battle. Now, however, America stands as one of the leading researchers and has made some incredible breakthroughs in scientific research with cancer cells.

It wasn't until the 1930s when someone discovered that a simple change in diet could inhibit the growth of many cancerous cells. Known as "**alkaline therapy**" "(pH therapy), this diet provides you with an all-in-one cancer inhibitor. Researchers realized that a person with cancer had their pH levels lowered to 6.5 to 7.5 to make it easier for the cancer cells to grow. If you were careful about what foods you consumed, you could potentially alter the pH levels in your body. This might make it harder for cancer cells to reproduce.

A high acidic diet (lowering your pH level below 6.5) can effectively prevent the growth of cancer cells. Unfortunately, it also causes a lot of pain in cancer patients. Therefore, a high alkaline diet (raising pH levels above 7.5) can be used to help a cancer patient's body eliminate latent acidosis and increase pH levels.

The body immediately begins to send cancer cells into "self-destruct" mode and the death of them follows suit shortly thereafter. While this diet is not an official treatment, it can be seen as a possible method of remission for cancer.

## AN 80'S WEIGHT LOSS SOLUTION WITH A CANCER CURING SIDE EFFECT

**Grapefruit** is another "super fruit" on the list of cancer preventions. These fruits are so powerful that people who eat them every day were shown to have a decrease in risk of cancer by as much as 50%.

What's their secret? They're high in vitamin C, a natural anticancer vitamin. A healthy daily portion can give you enough vitamin C to inhibit the growth of cancer cells and add a protective layer around organs to prevent their future growth.

They also provide you with added dietary fiber that helps prevent colon and rectum cancer by adding a protective layer over it. Additionally, high fiber diets regulate the body and stimulate the colon and rectum, preventing the proliferation of further cancer cells.

But those aren't the only benefits you get from the fruit. Grapefruits contain carotenoids, an antioxidant that helps reduce inflammation and increase immune system function. And lastly, they also contain lycopene — another powerful anticancer antioxidant. In combination with other foods, grapefruit can be a staple in a healthy diet.

## EGYPT'S $31 BILLION CANCER DISCOVERY

Curcumin was described earlier as a component of turmeric, a spice native to India and other regions around the world. **Curcumin** alone has its own anticancer properties. You can even double the effect of the substance if you combine it with green tea.

Green tea contains a component known as epigallocatechin Gallate (**ECGC**) which is known for preventing and inhibiting cancer growth. When combined with curcumin, the results are magnified. Curcumin allows the body to absorb a significantly larger portion of ECGC when it enters the body.

Curcumin and the high availability of ECGC helps reduce the risk of cancer by preventing the DNA replication process of cancerous cells. Cancer cells rely heavily on this process to grow quickly in the body. However, stopping this DNA replication can cause cancer cells to destroy itself due to improper DNA replication.

## THE ONLY CANCER TEST YOU SHOULD EVER TAKE

Every so often, life throws you a curveball. Something you can never really prepare for. Sometimes, it's something as harmless as a fender bender on your way to work. But in the worst case scenarios, it could be something as bad as cancer. You can take measures to try to protect yourself from it, but life doesn't always work out that way.

Luckily, there's a test you can take that might give you an early head's up. It's called **ONCOblot**, and it's an early cancer detection kid. What makes this kit stand out from other competitors on the market is that it can detect certain cancers before clinical symptoms appear. For example, it focuses on things called ENOX2 markers. These are specific protein species in the blood produced by malignant cancerous cells. The test helps eliminate false-positives that other medical tests might give you.

Just a head's up. You're going to need a physician to prescribe ONCOblot for you. But this one test could detect up to 10 types of cancerous cells. But even better than the money you could save is knowing you could detect a possible cancer early on.

## THE ONE CANCER TEST YOU SHOULD AVOID

You might want to hold off on your next prostate exam, even if your doctor recommends it. Most health insurance plans cover it, and it's recommended for men over the age of 40. But there's some things you need to consider before you do it.

There are certain things your doctor may not tell you prior to the test. Things you should ask about before you agree to anything. First, did you know there's an 80% chance the test will come back as a false-positive. Imagine all the added stress and panic you'll endure for a test that is wrong four out of five times.

Additionally, finding out you have cancer from a prostate test might not improve your chances anyway. The cancer grows very slowly and it's nearly impossible to detect.

You might want to consider taking an ONCOblot test. It's less invasive and more accurate.

**Women may also want to be careful about mammogram screenings. A recent study done in the U.K. showed that some women may have had unnecessary treatment for cancers that were unlikely to kill them or spread.**

## THE LASER LIGHT CANCER SOLUTION

Destroying cancer cells in the body should always be a top priority. Today, you could try a number of natural remedies or you can turn to modern medicine and technology. One modern option is **photodynamic therapy**.

This technology uses nontoxic light-sensitive drugs to target specific diseased cells. Next, a specially designed laser targets the drug, altering it and making it toxic to targeted cells. This option is popular amongst people who suffer throat or oral cancer.

This method can target and destroy precancerous and cancerous cells without damaging normal tissue. Chemotherapy and other cancer treatments can destroy malignant cells in the body, but are known to do significant damage to surrounding tissues and organs.

# CHAPTER 2: HEART DISEASE CURES

The next biggest killer of Americans is heart disease. This includes heart attacks and strokes. Each year, about 1.5 million Americans suffer heart attacks and strokes.

Put another way, daily, 2,200 people die from cardiovascular diseases. Every 44 seconds someone in the U.S. has a heart attack. And every 4 minutes, someone dies of a stroke.

Many people don't realize this but heart disease and stroke if survived, still can destroy your life because it can result in serious illness or disabilities.

It's an enormous problem that will affect almost every family. But if the FDA really had our interests at heart, then why are there so many people struggling with heart disease in our civilized, 1st world nation that flaunts it's amazing technology?

If you've paid attention to the FDA's food pyramid, you'll notice it's always suggested a low fat diet with a huge emphasis on grains and carbohydrates. Meat also took a backseat in regards to what foods should be emphasized.

So for decades now, most people have had it hammered into their heads that a high fiber, low fat diet is the healthiest diet there is. The epidemic increase in heart disease proves otherwise. You see, what the FDA's food pyramid suggests as science is actually not sound science.

It all goes back to the research conducted by Ancel Keys and his seven countries study which tracked the fat consumption and heart disease levels of various nations. It was named for seven specific countries that saw an increase in heart disease cases that seemed to correspond with increased fat consumption.

But in reality, it should have been named the 22 countries study because he deliberately omitted lots of data that was counter to his conclusion that a low fat, low protein diet is necessary to reduce heart disease.

The FDA used this faulty study to shape the diet plan of Americans and of course, food companies went along with it producing low fat and high fiber products. Year after year, this concept of heart healthy has been layered into the thinking of Americans.

And yet, heart disease is neck and neck with cancer as the leading killer in America. Go figure.

It's certainly true that some fats are healthier than others. Trans-fats are poison for your arteries. Fortunately many efforts are in place to strip it out of our foods.

Back to our story: Some people believe there was a deliberate reasoning behind this faulty diet plan.

To create plenty of new cases of heart disease to be treated by big corporations. Others feel, the big push towards a low protein diet is for the purpose of creating a more apathetic populace. Often you'll find in a cult that they serve low fat, low protein meals to make it easier to control their cult members.

On that same note, your brain is made of fat, and requires fat to properly function. If you're not getting enough healthy fats, then your brain performance suffers. Just something to think about.

## 4 STEPS TOWARDS A HEALTHY HEART

Poor food choices, high levels of sugar, and stress damage the body in the short run and have lasting effects in the long run, especially on your heart. And a healthy heart is the first step towards a healthier and longer life. Changing your diet today to strengthen and protect your heart could mean an extra 10 years in your life.

There are certain food restrictions and life changes you need to be aware of. Here are a few pointers.

- Eat More Salt — Though it might go against popular opinion, your body actually does need a healthy amount of salt to survive. Studies have shown diets with low salt intake were more likely to have higher mortality rates than diets with moderate salt intake. Long term salt deprivation could have serious negative consequences on your body.

- Get Married — It might surprise you, but having someone to share the rest of your life with could actually improve your health. Studies have shown that married men and women enjoy a better quality of life. Those who are happy in their marriage also have a 46% lower rate of mortality compared to single people.

- Have More Sex — Sex is actually great for your health. It's part of human nature and it can actually help reduce heart problems. Men who say they have sex at least twice a week are significantly healthier and are less likely to suffer from a heart attack. It also helps lower blood pressure, reduce stress, and even keep you emotionally healthy.

- Drink Alcohol — Drinking in moderation can actually be good for you. Studies have shown a drink or two can reduce the chance of heart disease in men. In fact, one study showed that light, moderate, and even heavy drinkers could reduce their chance of heart disease by 35%, 51%, and 54%, respectively. Though we don't recommend you become a heavy drinker because of the other negative consequences that go along with that. That being said, don't feel too guilty the next time you go out and have some drinks with your friends.

---

**If you need more convincing that salt is actually good for you, here's some more information. The government was wrong when they said low sodium diets were good for you. They even tried to link salt to problems like high blood pressure and heart disease, though new studies have proven that false. In fact, low sodium diets have been linked with higher instances of insulin resistance. Consider natural salt options like sea salt when looking to add it into your diet.**

---

## PROTECT YOUR HEART WITH THIS 15 MINUTE EXERCISE

A lot of people refer to LDL cholesterol as "bad cholesterol" and many people blame it for a number of heart related problems. But when people have a heart attack only about half of them have high LDL cholesterol levels.

LDL cholesterol still plays a major part in many heart attacks. But new research is pointing to high blood pressure as having a bigger role. High blood pressure puts added pressure on the heart and causes it to work at high rates for an extended amount of time. This causes blood to pump through your system faster. Unless you take control of your high blood pressure now, you could be at risk of suffering a serious heart attack.

It's recommended that you take blood pressure medication to prevent a heart attack within the first 15-minutes of experiencing high blood pressure. This is the only "bullet proof" method of ridding high blood pressure quickly.

---

**If you have the money, think about investing in a blood pressure machine. You can keep an eye on your blood pressure without having to see your doctor constantly. You can pick up a unit at an online retailers like Amazon for around $50.**

---

## THE FRENCH PARADOX HEART SOLUTION

Studies have shown French people have a diet just as unhealthy as Americans. They also have high rates of smoking and drinking. So why is it the French are 50% less likely to suffer from a heart attack than an American?

France and America don't see eye to eye when it comes to what they do in their downtime. Americans are normally hard working, and see rest and relaxation as something you do after you finish a day's work. The French, on the other hand, see things differently.

The average Frenchmen take their jobs seriously, but they also take their time-off just as serious. Long leisurely lunches, frequent naps, and vacations help relax their mind and body. This lessens the tension in the body and reduces stress. It also gives their bodies adequate time to rest. Invest in longer lunches, napping a bit more and schedule your next vacation to remove stress and add fun to your life. Doing this lessens the risk of heart disease!

---

**If you happen to be out for a nice leisurely stroll during the summer, consider getting yourself a smoothie made with whole milk. The high levels of vitamin D will decrease your chances of developing heart disease.**

---

## THE $1.99 HYPERTENSION AND CHOLESTEROL SOLUTION

Eating **garlic** has been proven to help with your heart health. This simple seasoning has multiple purposes and many people swear by it. However, if you knew it could save your heart, would you eat it more often?

Garlic gives you access to an abundance of vitamins and minerals that can keep you healthy. When you eat it, you ingest a powerful compound called "allicin." This compound helps lower blood pressure to healthy levels. People who ate more garlic saw up to an 8% reduction in blood pressure.

Garlic is even known for softening arteries. This helps people who have limited flexibility and mobility. High levels of stress can lead to atherosclerosis, which may increase the possibility of a heart attack due to the strain on your body. Garlic reduces this risk by promoting flexibility and mobility. Lastly, studies have also shown garlic helps lower LDL cholesterol levels.

## A MEXICAN "SUPER FOOD" THAT CAN STRENGTHEN YOUR HEART

**Avocados** are categorized as a "super food" and, often times, have multiple uses for curing diseases. Earlier you read about how avocados contained special compounds that reduce the risk of cancer. But they do more than just that. They also help reduce the chances of heart disease.

Avocados are a great food for your heart. They're low in trans-fat, saturated fat, cholesterol, and sodium. On top of all that, avocados help your body generally function better. They contain monosaturated fats, which lowers LDL (bad) cholesterol while promoting HDL (good) cholesterol.

There are plenty of ways you can incorporate it into your diet. Add it to a sandwich or use it to make guacamole. For an even tastier and healthier treat, add tomatoes and onions to your guacamole and top it off with some lime juice.

## IT'S FINALLY OK TO EAT CHOCOLATE!

Commonly found in chocolate, **vitamin D** does more than provide your body with necessary nutrients; it also can help reduce certain diseases, especially heart disease.

Unlike other vitamins, vitamin D has long-term health benefits. When you lack this vitamin, your skin begins to deteriorate, causing your complexion to fade. It may even cause your skin to wrinkle.

Making sure you have enough vitamin D in your system every day will give you a healthier body in no time. When taking vitamin D, you're able to prevent immune disorders, diabetes, and osteoarthritis. Vitamin D can even regulate your heart and prevent it from going into "overdrive" when facing stress or strain.

## STOP BLAMING SALT! THE REAL CULPRIT BEHIND YOUR HIGH BLOOD PRESSURE

**Stress** is one of the biggest reasons why so many people have heart disease. When you're faced with a lot of stress, your body goes into overdrive.

One way your body changes during stressful times is by raising its blood pressure. Pumping more blood can make your body wake itself up and can send adrenaline rushing through your system. You might think this sounds like a good thing, but it also increases your chance of having a heart attack.

Heart problems are often associated with high levels of stress. Anything above normal blood pressure could alter your eating habits and lead you to an unhealthy diet. Stress brings on sugar cravings that can spike your insulin levels. Once those levels spike, your blood pressure may increase for a short amount of time. It's during this time when a heart attack may incur.

Reducing stress may be the single important aspect of your treatment for heart disease. Yoga and pilates are excellent ways to get it under control. In fact, any moderate exercise is good for you in the long run.

## THE CENTRAL AMERICAN HYPERTENSION KILLER

Do you consume enough **vitamin D3** in your diet? The recommended daily value of vitamin D is 200 IU for any adult under the age of 50, 400 for adults 51–70 and 600 IU for adults over 70. But why does the recommended value of the vitamin increase as we age?

As our bodies get older, they begin to deteriorate. So it's important to listen to your body and not to overexert yourself. In fact, if you are overly active, increasing your vitamin D3 intake is a must.

Vitamin D3 is known as a cholecalciferol and it's a vitamin obtained in a synthetic form such as a pill. This vitamin is able to increase the amount of "good" cholesterol ("HDL Cholesterol") in your body. The more good cholesterol you have, the better. It also regulates the heart and protects it from high blood pressure.

## THE HEALTHY HEART SECRET BURIED WITH THE ANCIENT MUMMIES

While not all seafood may be "heart healthy," certain fish such as salmon and mackerel contain a vital nutrient for assisting with heart health. **Omega-3** and **omega-6 fatty acids** derive from the natural oil fish produce. They're even available over-the-counter at your local pharmacy.

Research has shown that omega-3 fatty acids lower both blood pressure and triglycerine levels. Lowered levels of triglycerine and blood pressure help reduce the risk of heart attacks, strokes and even death from heart disease. Even further, you can lessen the painful symptoms of rheumatoid arthritis.

Take fish oil capsules if you are unable to eat enough fish. If you are vegetarian or vegan, flaxseed is a good alternative. They're slightly different, but still just as effective. And, of course, you could get your fill by substituting one of your weekly meals with fish.

---

**Did you know krill oil can also protect your skin from damage caused by the sun?**

---

## STOP BLOOD CLOTS BEFORE THEY EVEN FORM

**Flavonoid** is a basic compound found in many fruits and vegetables. However, what really makes flavonoid unique and healthy is a compound found inside of it. This compound is commonly known as "**rutin**." Because Americans often consume not enough flavonoid, we usually don't consume a healthy amount of rutin. In fact, American diets lack this nutrient so much that some scientists suspect this could be why the number one cause of death in the U.S. is heart disease and stroke. A simple change in your diet can affect your lifespan and way of life.

Found inside our cells is a substance called, "protein disulfide isomerase ("PDI"). All animals secrete this substance. This protein could create something called a thrombosis, a potentially fatal blot clot. However, consuming fruits and vegetables rich in flavonoid could decrease the chance of a thrombosis forming. Consuming more fruits and vegetables will increase the amount of flavonoid in your body, which will decrease the risk of other heart related ailments.

Instead of taking a potentially dangerous blood thinner that could cause menstrual bleeding, red or brown urine, or could make your bowel movements look like tar, consider eating foods high in flavonoid rutin. These include: apples, onions, citrus fruits, asparagus.

## THE "GLASS HALF FULL" HEALTH SOLUTION

Reducing stress is one method of reducing heart disease. In addition to removing stress, your way of thinking also affects the health of your heart. Studies have shown that people who have a more positive outlook on life decrease their chances of illnesses and other dangers.

What makes the power of thought so important to heart health?

It's all about how you look at life. Naturally, your body will act accordingly. The more negative you think, the more that negatively affects your body. This can cause unnecessary stress and, in addition, high blood pressure.

**Positive thinking** can do the opposite.

In addition, many diseases only become fatal if you believe they will be. The mind has a lot of power over the way our body reacts. So clear your mind, become a more optimistic person, look at the glass half full, and you could possibly save yourself from a life-threatening heart attack.

## WHIP UP A BATCH OF "HYPERTENSION SOUP"

**Gazpacho soup** is a traditional cold tomato soup that origin in Spain but is common in many Mediterranean dishes. What mak gazpacho soup so beneficial is that it's made up of six super foods: tomatoes, cucumber, bell peppers, olive oil, onions and garlic.

Garlic is a known preventive for heart attacks by reducing blood pressure. There is a special ingredient named "allinin" which helps with reduce blood pressure. Tomatoes are high in lycopene and help reduce heart disease. This antioxidant assists with lowering blood pressure significantly and can help reduce clogs in your arteries.

In combination with the other vegetables, gazpacho is filled with flavonoids, containing the compound rutin. Rutin is known for preventing heart attacks by reducing the amount of a certain protein developed within the body. Even further, it helps reduce the risk of blood clots by thinning the blood.

## THE SLEEP HEALTH HACK TO ENSURE YOU WAKE UP TOMORROW

**Water** is a solution for many problems. Which makes sense since it's an essential part of life. No other liquid can be consumed at such high levels the way water can be consumed.

Consuming water does more than just hydrate your body. It can also help with basic bodily functions like improving blood flow. Consistent water intake will help your body naturally thin your blood as opposed to taking a life-threatening blood thinner.

Thicker blood takes more time to process through the blood stream. If you decide to increase water how much water you drink, you can potentially reduce the risk of clogged arteries. Drink a few more glasses of water a day and you can decrease your rate of a heart attack as much as 50%.

---

**Water might be a great natural sleep remedy, but don't go overboard drinking it. In fact, the old advice saying you should drink at least eight cups of water a day could be detrimental to your health. Why? Because too much water throws off the electrolyte balance in your body. Drinking water to cleanse your body of harmful toxins is great... to a point. Too much water might rid your body of essential minerals, disrupting your body's natural chemical balance. This could lead to water intoxication with symptoms like headaches, drowsiness, and irritability.**

---

**…nake sure you're drinking and using the cleanest water …a whole house filter. Check out waterfilers.mercola.com …v you can get your hands on one.**

## …ISTAN'S HIDDEN HEART CURE

The Hunza are a group of people who live in the Himalayan Mountains in Pakistan. These people have been living nearly disease-free for hundreds of years and some of them are well over 100 years old. What makes them even more spectacular is that they do not use a lot of modern medicine. In fact, they mainly use natural remedies.

One main reason behind their health and longevity is the food they eat, in particular their traditional **Hunza bread**. It accompanies practically every meal. The grain is preserved and matured for as long as possible and they only grind as much as they need for each meal. This grain provides the people with tasty bread that does not go bad. In addition, the grain is great for your heart since it reduces stress by slowing and regulating blood flow.

---

**Hunza Bread isn't the only cure originating in the Himalayans. The Ayuvedic herb known as Bacopa sharpens your brain, improves memory, and enhances cognitive function. You can purchase the herb in caplet form.**

---

## THE 60 SECOND HEART ATTACK STOPPER

Heart attacks are one of the most common heart disease cases in America. It happens often due to a combination of high stress levels, blocked arteries and high cholesterol. The most common symptom of an incoming heart attack is tingling or pain in your left arm. However, did you know you could stop that right in its tracks?

**Cayenne pepper** is one of the most uncommon saviors in stopping a heart attack. Capsaicin, an active component in cayenne pepper, helps stimulate warm circulation in blood. This stimulates the heart and arteries, giving your body the ability to return to normal.

It takes less than 60 seconds for the effects of cayenne pepper to set in. If you think you or someone you know might be having a heart attack, mix one teaspoon of cayenne pepper in warm water. Drink it immediately before you lose consciousness. Hopefully, in less than a minute, the heart attack will go away.

---

**As if preventing a heart attack isn't a good enough reason to keep the pepper permanently stocked in your house, it could also help reduce LDL cholesterol in your system.**

---

## THE ONE FOOD YOU CAN EAT TO "TURN OFF" HEART DISEASE

Beetroots, spinach, celery, radishes and lettuces have the most amount of healthy dietary nitrates available. Stick within this range and it will help you find cures to diseases such as heart disease and diabetes. Dietary nitrates possess a compound known as nitric oxide, which assists in maintaining a molecules' contractility and strengthens vascular smooth muscle cells. Nitric oxide has been linked to improving vascular health and preventing the proliferation of cells in the heart.

Many **leafy greens** also contain flavonoid rutin and vitamin D. These help maintain a healthy heart. Additionally, both of these vitamins and minerals can naturally thin your blood, decreasing your chance of contracting a blood clot. Leafy greens should be eaten on a daily basis for the nutrients they contain.

## WHY YOU SHOULD STICK TO THE ORIGINAL WHITE MEAT

Vegetarians and vegans might miss out on this next solution. Eating meats other than **chicken** could be more hazardous for your health. Fats and high levels of salt in traditional meats like pork clog arteries and could lead to other health problems. Once they're clogged, blood clots begin to form and it could results in a backwards flow of blood. This could cause the heart to speed up rapidly and may result in a greater chance of a heart attack.

Eating chicken could prevent all this. It's low in sodium, carbs and fats, and the meat is lean, making it easier for you to digest.

## DON'T FEEL GUILTY ABOUT ORDERING THAT STEAK

**Red meat**'s gotten a bad rap over the years. It's been blamed as contributing to heart disease, cancer, and it's even been accused of speeding up aging. But people who make these claims aren't presenting all the facts.

For example, if you have an active lifestyle the negative effects of red meat are not as pronounced. Sedentary and inactive lifestyles exacerbate the problems brought on by red meat. If you're burning a high number of calories every day through daily exercising, you'll absorb more protein from red meat and mitigate the negative side effects.

Just look at any bodybuilder or athlete. For many of them, red meat and other high protein meats are a main part of their diets. Half a pound of red meat has up to 15mg of vitamin B3, also known as niacin. This substance aids with digestion, helps production of good cholesterol, and expands and dilates blood vessels.

Also, remember not to overcook your meat. Cooking it to medium will maximize its health potential and decrease your risk of developing certain cancers.

Additionally, red meat is an excellent source of zinc, iron, and selenium. Zinc increases sperm count in men, and helps keep the prostate healthy. Overall, red meats helps increase oxygen levels in the blood stream, lowers the chance of developing heart problems, and can even boost the immune system. But remember, you'll need to maintain an active lifestyle to enjoy these positive benefits.

---

**Speaking of selenium, did you know diets high in the substance have been known to have lower instances of some forms of cancers. One study showed that Japanese and Bulgarian diets, known for their high levels of selenium, produced lower instances of mammary tumors in mice.**

---

## YOUR VEGETARIAN FRIENDS ARE WRONG

The next time your vegetarian friend tries to make you feel guilty because you ordered a steak, tell him to calm down. His vegetarian lifestyle might not offer all the health benefits he thinks it does. In fact, there might not be any life expectancy advantages from removing meat from your diet.

Eating fruits and vegetables along with grains, dairy, and eggs provides you with many necessary nutrients. But that still doesn't overcome the nutrients lost by forgoing meat. A healthy active life-style along with a diet with healthy proportions of meat can improve life expectancy. Skipping out on the meat might save you money, but it won't save you the years of your life.

## CHECK YOURSELF FOR THIS HEART RISK FACTOR IMMEDIATELY

The next time you see your doctor, ask him to make sure the level of **homocysteine** in your body is normal. High concentrations of this amino acid could indicate a higher risk of having a stroke or a heart attack. If you have a family history of heart disease, but do not have any other obvious risk factors, it might be a good idea to ask for this test.

# CHAPTER 3: CHOLESTEROL CURES

For most people over 50, when they get a checkup, the big barometer of heart health seems to be their LDL cholesterol, in relation to their triglicerides, and their HDL cholesterol. Conventional medicine suggests you've got to watch your bad cholesterol like a hawk and gulp down pills to get it into the right ratio.

For many people whose cholesterol is out of ratio, they often get talked into taking cholesterol drugs called Statins.

Statins come with a dirty laundry list of problems.

That's because not only do they inhibit production of cholesterol, they interfere with other intermediary substances which have important biochemical functions.

One of which is they deplete the body of Coenzyme Q10 (CoQ10) which is vital to heart health and muscle function.

Most doctors aren't really up to speed on the true dangers of Statins. Too many times, patients came down with fatigue, muscle weakness, soreness, and in some cases, heart failure. Statin drugs are also linked to:

- Nerve damage in the hands and feet.
- Dizzy spells.
- Memory loss.
- Higher cancer risk.
- Weakened immune system.
- Depression.
- Liver problems.

OK, fine. There are side effects. So are these drugs effective?

Let's look at Pfizer's Lipitor, which is the most prescribed cholesterol medication in the world and has been prescribed to more than 26 million Americans.

According to Lipitor's own Web site, Lipitor is proven to lower bad cholesterol 39–60 percent, depending on the dose. Sounds effective, right?

Well, *BusinessWeek* did an excellent story on this topic and they found the real numbers right on Pfizer's own newspaper ad for Lipitor.

Upon first glance, the ad claims Lipitor reduces heart attacks by 36 percent. But there's an asterisk. And when you follow that asterisk, you find the following in smaller type:

> *"That means in a large clinical study, 3% of patients taking a sugar pill or placebo had a heart attack compared to 2% of patients taking Lipitor."*

What this means is that for every 100 people who took the drug over 3.3 years, three people on placebos, and two people on Lipitor, had heart attacks.

So taking Lipitor resulted in just one fewer heart attack per 100 people.

This drug is barely more effective than the placebo!

But these aren't the only cholesterol lowering drugs being prescribed, there's Zetia and Vytorin among others.

Look — Mother Nature has solutions for your cholesterol. And her solutions definitely outperform placebos. Plus… they come with few if any side effects.

## VITAMIN "Q" — THE VITAMIN DRUG COMPANIES TRIED TO PATENT

**Coenzyme Q10 (CoQ10)** is a component found in every cell in the human body. The body naturally produces the substance and uses it to produce the energy your cells need for growth. Furthermore, the component is known to work as an antioxidant, protecting the body from damage. What makes this component unique is its ability to help reduce cholesterol levels in your body.

When you take a CoQ10 supplement, you'll immediately feel lighter on your feet and your body will be able to handle more damage.

However, before taking the supplement, make sure you tell your doctor. CoQ10 also seems to show signs of lowering cholesterol levels by acting as an antioxidant and removing bad molecules from the body, including LDL cholesterol.

## THE CHOLESTEROL KILLER THAT COULD HELP YOU LOSE WEIGHT

There are a number of foods that have such tremendous effects on the body we call them "super foods." **Macadamia oil** is one of those foods. This fat has been shown to assist with heart health.

Macadamia oil has one of the highest concentrations of monosaturated fats than any other oil. Monosaturated fats are "good fats" that help promote HDL Cholesterol (the good kind) in the body, while also lowering LDL cholesterol.

Macadamia oil has one of the most potent effects on the heart and can return your health from bad to good if you incorporate it into your diet. In addition to lowering LDL cholesterol, macadamia oil has high levels of oleic acid, which helps improve memory, reduces inflammation and increases testosterone levels.

---

**Speaking of nuts, check out coconut oil for a safe and healthy way to control your weight. It's anti-microbial, anti-histamine, and anti-diabetic. It's another miracle food you can only find in nature (and not in some scientist's lab). And if you really want to kick things up a notch, consider using coconut oil the next time you want fried food. It's a healthy alternative that adds incredible flavor to whatever meal you're making.**

---

## THE CHOLESTEROL CURE HIDING IN THE ASIAN FOOD SECTION

**Red yeast rice** is a traditional staple in Chinese medicine and has been proven to assist with lowering cholesterol levels. Difficult to come by, red yeast rice is now sold in over-the-counter supplements at your pharmacy or local grocery store. While sometimes inconvenient to get, the benefits make purchasing the supplement a necessity for improved heart health.

Red yeast rice has been shown to reduce cholesterol levels. When a patient took 2.4 grams of red yeast rice per day, it reduced their LDL levels an average of 22%. Overall, you could expect to see a decrease in cholesterol of around 16% after 12 weeks. Red yeast rice covers your body with a lining that prevents LDL cholesterol from being absorbed excessively through the blood stream and potentially causing a blocked artery.

On average, the recommended value of red yeast rice you should digest daily is between 1.3 to 2.4 grams per day. This will help the body remove LDL cholesterol over time, improving heart function.

---

**Just a word of warning when it comes to supplements. Make sure you don't overdo it. Supplements can be a great way to get important nutrients into your body, but going overboard can be disastrous (and it might lead to a number of eye problems). Follow the instructions and consult a professional who understands your personal health needs, if possible.**

---

## A REVOLUTIONARY WAY OF REMOVING POISONS FROM YOUR BODY

**Chelation therapy** is an alternative medical technique that involves administering specific substances to reduce and remove heavy metals from your body. This kind of therapy is very effective in removing certain toxins and poisons, such as lead and arsenic, that might have found their way into your body.

The process involves injecting the synthetic solution ethylenediaminetetraacetic acid (EDTA) into your body. It then bonds with harmful heavy metals and makes it easier for your body to flush out the poison safely. It's believed that EDTA acts like an antioxidant and helps promote and protect your body's immune system.

Some health officials also believe chelation therapy can be used to attach and remove LDL cholesterol from your system. People have also reported less pain and complications from diseases and ailments such as lupus, arthritis and scleroderma.

Care should be taken when considering chelation therapy. Thorough research, as well as approval from your doctor, should be taken before you decide to undergo this treatment option.

# CHAPTER 4: DIABETES

Today, diabetes affects 25.8 million people in the United States. That's three times the size of the population of Austria. And some 7 million people are estimated to have diabetes but aren't diagnosed, that's almost twice the population of Ireland.

Many people don't realize just how serious diabetes can be. It's the leading cause of kidney failure and non-traumatic lower-limb amputations and new cases of blindness.

It's also a major cause of heart disease and stroke.

It's predicted that by 2050, 20% to 30% of the U.S. population will have diabetes. United Healthcare estimates that over the next decade, the United States will spend a staggering $3.4 trillion in costs due to diabetes.

With all of the drugs out there, why aren't things getting better?

When the drug industry spends an outrageous 19 times more on self-promotion than on research, you know the answer. There's more money to be made in treating the illness than in curing it.

Just listen to what happened with the popular drug Avandia. This one's a doozy. This drug hit the market in 1999 after a multi-million dollar advertising campaign. Seven years later, it brought in $3.2 billion a year in revenue.

What are the chances some VIPs got million dollar bonuses over that.

But then in 2009, sales dropped $1.2 billion after a study published in *The New England Journal of Medicine* linked Avandia to a 43 percent increased risk of heart attack and a 64 percent higher risk of cardiovascular death. This should have shut the drug down right there, don't you agree?

It didn't! The FDA oversight board held a vote and decided to keep the drug on the market.

This isn't one isolated case. This is par for the course my friend.

By some estimations, drugs like Vioxx have been estimated to have killed thousands of unsuspecting patients. But check this out. It get even crazier…

The Mayo Clinic a few years back recommended a new software that shows a patient when he should begin taking Statin drugs to offset heart disease risks. Did you see that?

It's a sneaky way of tricking unsuspecting patients into getting on Statin drugs. So now this patient is juggling two drug prescriptions. That's twice the revenue stream.

It's a crazy world we live in.

Ok, but there's good news. Mother Nature again has cures waiting in the wings — even for diabetes. If only we'd just listen to her.

## A DIABETIC'S WONDER TEA

This beverage is popular in South Africa since the **redbush tea tree** is native to the country. The tea is created by fermenting, or "oxidizing," the leaves. This fermented process gives the tea a pungent taste that is enjoyable to many. It even has antioxidants that assist with diabetes.

Redbush tea has been shown to metabolize fats quicker in the body. Along with a well-balanced diet and some exercising, you can easily shed pounds off your body, reducing the chances of having diabetes as your body begins functioning better.

For those with long-term diabetes, when taken as a supplement in controlled dosages, redbush tea was able to positively affect hypoglycemic levels. It can be taken orally through a supplement form and can help stabilize your sugar levels promptly.

---

**Since we're talking about antioxidants, you should know there's another popular (and delicious) food chock full of the stuff that can also help you lose weight. Shockingly, it's butter. Avoid margarine or other alternative stuffed with chemicals. Make sure the butter you buy is made with milk from grass-fed cows and you should be alright.**

---

## THE CHINESE "BEAN CURE" YOU PROBABLY ALREADY EAT

The controversy surrounding the health benefits of **soy** has been debated for decades. The underlying fact is that soy does contain certain health benefits that are great for overall body function. Taking soy in moderation is suggestible, and can be especially beneficial if you're diabetic.

Soy products like tempeh and tofu are great options if you don't know where to start. Soy foods are low on the glycemic index and are excellent sources of fiber. These foods may improve insulin production in your body and regulate your blood sugar level. In addition, soy has been shown to help protect the kidney in diabetes patients.

Furthermore, soy is low in calories and has high nutritional value. When eaten in moderation along with other healthy foods, it can reduce the amount of fat, calories, and cholesterol you consume and help mitigate diabetes symptoms.

## THE DIABETES CURE YOU CAN BUY AT WAL-MART

Diets rich in sugars not only could lead to Type II Diabetes, they could also promote the growth of certain tumors. People with diabetes could see a drastic improvement in their health by consuming a substance called **nicotinamide mononucleotide** (NMN, for short).

When your body digests and breaks down NMN, it enhances your hepatic insulin sensitivity. In other words, it helps regulates the spikes and drops in sugar in your body. Additionally, after you consume a large enough amount of NMN, your body will begin to restore nutrients that also assist with restoring gene expression.

If you've found it difficult in keeping your diabetes under control, seeking medical attention should be your first priority. Sudden drops or spikes in your blood sugar can be temporarily fixed with NMN until you reach proper medical attention.

## THE NEW EUROPEAN DIET PERFECT FOR DIABETICS

A new "craze" known as the "**Mediterranean Diet**" has hit the market. This diet is rich in fish, beans, fruits, vegetables, olive oil and nuts. It also limits how much dairy you should consume and allows moderate alcohol consumption. However, people don't complain because they're thankful for a diet that actually allows you to have a beer or a glass of wine every now and then.

When studying a random list of people aged 55 to 80 (the primary age range of diabetics) people who ate the Mediterranean diet were less likely to get diabetes. When taking a Mediterranean diet supplemented with olive oil, it reduced the risk of diabetes by 40%. Adding nuts to the diet had an 18% reduction.

Also, make sure the olive oil you're buying is pure. Read the fine print on the bottle and make sure the bottle was packaged in Italy and that it isn't mixed with other oils.

These foods help stimulate insulin production and aid the pancreas by keeping levels from spiking or dropping drastically.

---

**Speaking of alcohol, did you know there's one type of drink you can get at the bar that might improve your chances against cancer. We're talking about scotch. Single malt, in fact, since it has high levels of ellagic acid, a powerful antioxidant against certain cancers. And don't feel guilty about having a couple of beers after work. A glass or two a day can flood your body with powerful antioxidants, aid in your digestion, and even decrease stress and strengthen your heart.**

---

## THE BEST EXERCISES TO FIGHT AGAINST DIABETES

Of all possible cures, exercise has the highest success rate of curing Type II diabetes and reducing the symptoms in Type I diabetes patients.

When you begin exercising, you immediately help your body process the glucose it needs and pump it straight into your bloodstream. Once you begin sweating, you are able to reduce blood glucose by excreting the insulin through your pores. When you exercise more, you are able to keep your insulin levels consistent. If your glucose levels spike, a quick run can help reduce it immediately.

Never forget to regulate your blood sugar with healthy foods and activity. The more you exercise, the more you'll have to consume certain sugars. Before beginning any new exercise regimen, make sure you talk to your doctor. Your physician will be able to provide you with all the necessary information to get your diabetes under control.

Consider purchasing a set of resistance bands and doing a variety of resistance based workouts. You can buy a set online for roughly $30.

## BEST FOODS TO LOWER BLOOD SUGAR

Controlling your blood sugar levels is the best thing you can do to mitigate the negative effects and symptoms of diabetes. And the best way to do that is to be aware of the foods and substances you put in your body. Here's a list of the best foods someone with diabetes could eat to maintain a healthy diet. Incorporate five of these foods into your diet for 6 weeks and your doctor will be amazed at the level of improvement you'll achieve.

### Whole-Fat Dairy

Make sure you get three to five servings of whole fat dairy products like milk, yogurt and cheese. Trans-palmitoleic acid found in this type of food helps regulate the body's blood sugar.

### Vinegar

Two to three tablespoons of vinegar before or with a meal can reduce sugar levels between 25–50%.

### Chocolate

This should be great news to any chocolate lovers out there. Three ounces of dark chocolate can reduce insulin sensitivity in your body if consumed daily. This type of chocolate has been shown to accelerate the body's ability to process and metabolize glucose in the body.

### Apples

Apples are known for having high levels of quercetin. The higher the levels of quercetin, the more potent the effects. Apples have shown to reduce the risk of diabetes by as much as 20%.

### Garlic

Garlic helps regulate the body's insulin levels and helps prevent spikes or drops in your blood levels. Even better, garlic can help with low blood sugar by promoting insulin production. Two to three cloves a day is more than enough for the average person.

### Green Tea

Regulating blood sugar has never been easier than with green tea. This tea has an abundance of antioxidants that assists with producing insulin, regulating it and helping the body metabolize glucose. Two to three cups daily will show the most beneficial results.

### Cinnamon

Ingesting cinnamon has an abundance of positive health benefits for you. A daily diet with at least half a teaspoon of cinnamon can help lower sugar levels by as much as 8%.

---

**Did you know the last place you want to look to help manage your diabetes is the FDA's official Food Pyramid. Why? They tell you to load up the base of your diet with grains, pastas and breads. These carbohydrates are just another way to introduce sugars into your system. The Food Pyramid looks more like a favor to special interest groups than it does sound nutritional advice.**

---

## ANOTHER BIBLICAL HEALTH CURE

**Holy thorn** is one of those plants you rarely hear about unless there is something wrong with your body. Native to China, you can now get this plant in over-the-counter supplements. Being used as a traditional remedy in Chinese medicine for over 1,400 years, this product can aid with controlling glucose levels.

When consuming holy thorn extract, you'll begin to feel its effects immediately. The product helps stimulate your body's pancreas and will help keep blood sugar levels at normal levels. Furthermore, the plant is able to improve A1C levels, which help regulate insulin in your body. You can properly maintain your body with this supplement by reducing sugar spikes and increasing insulin sensitivity.

## STOP SUGAR SPIKES IN THEIR TRACKS

You might have heard of **chromium** being used in cars and in construction projects. But did you know this metal is essential to maintaining a healthy diet. Also known as an "essential trace element," it provides diabetics with a wide number of benefits.

When consuming chromium picolinate orally, a person can quickly reduce their high blood sugar. This substance assists the body by reducing blood sugar, reducing insulin levels and even assisting with insulin production for some diabetics.

Additionally, this trace element is found in many diabetic medicines. When consumed, it helps reduce fat intake and can also help by preventing weight gain. In fact, this has been shown to help with weight loss.

## THE CINNAMON AND HONEY BIBLE CURE

History is filled with major breakthroughs in medicine. Some of the best discoveries come from eastern medicines and remedies that use fewer chemicals and more organic substances. A recent breakthrough in major eastern medicine is the new "Bible Cure" for diabetes. This cure is a combination of **cinnamon** and **honey**.

Honey is beneficial for the body, especially when eaten in its raw form. It's the only food that never spoils or rots. This allowed many people to store and use it later. In traditional eastern medicine, honey is an ideal supplement because of this particular benefit. When combined with cinnamon, it will help improve your body's overall health.

Cinnamon and honey act as a repellent for bad molecules and are filled with hundreds of live molecules that assist with the digestion process. When entering the body, the cinnamon and honey stick against the lining of the stomach and intestine. This helps reduce the amount of insulin absorbed into the blood stream, preventing insulin spikes from occurring.

The benefits of cinnamon and honey are abundant. The more you consume, the better your health will be long-term. You can help control diabetes with this simple recipe. Combine one part honey, one part cinnamon, and ten parts water.

## THE BEST DIABETIC SUPPLEMENTS TO TAKE

Diabetes hinders the way the body metabolizes glucose. While healthy eating and daily exercise is probably the best way to reduce sugar spikes and blood sugar drops, taking supplements can also help.

Listed below are supplements that will mitigate symptoms associated with diabetes by making your body more insulin-sensitive. Additionally, these supplements slow down your body's ability to absorb sugars and fats. Healthy levels of cholesterol and blood sugar give diabetics more energy, fewer sugar cravings and help with weight maintenance.

- Vitamin D3 — 1,000 to 2,000 IU with breakfast
- Cinnamon — 125 mg to 150mg
- Fish Oil — 1,000 to 2,000 mg.
- Magnesium — 100 mg to 200 mg.
- Chromium Polynicotinate — 100 to 300 mcg
- Multivitamin — As directed
- Green Tea Catechins — 25 to 50 mg
- Biotin — 1 to 2 mg.
- Alpha Lipoic Acid — 300 to 600 mg.
- PGX — 2.5g before every meal

---

**Regardless of what natural remedy or cure you decide to try in your fight against diabetes, here are three simple tips that can help you: 1. Stop drinking sugary drinks and sodas. 2. Exercise daily. It might hurt in the beginning, but it's worth it in the end. 3. Watch your diet. Your body functions off the food you give it. Remember that every time you eat something unhealthy.**

---

# CHAPTER 5: PAIN CURES

The next health problem that hits home for a lot of people is chronic pain. Based upon the findings of a report from the Institute of Medicine, more than 100 million Americans suffer from chronic pain at a cost of around $60 billion a year in medical treatments and lost productivity.

Surprisingly, that number is expected to rise higher as baby boomers age. That being the case, by 2030, 40 percent of American adults will suffer some sort of arthritic disease.

Wait, how can this be? The FDA and big pharma claim their approved solutions are the only legitimate way to treat pain problems. These guys are like professional con artists.

Here's something these guys hope you don't ever find out…

Today, prescription drugs are the second-most abused category of drugs in the nation. Prescription painkillers are a major contributor to the total number of drug deaths in the country.

And the estimated number of emergency department visits linked to non-medical drug use of pain relievers nearly doubled between 2004 and 2009.

Addiction cases are growing. In 2010, about 12 million Americans age 12 and older admit non-medical use of prescription painkillers in the past year. This probably includes painkillers like OxyContin.

Ok, many people feel they get some benefit from painkillers. Fair enough. But the opiate kind, the high powered stuff can cause addiction. Trust me, you don't want that.

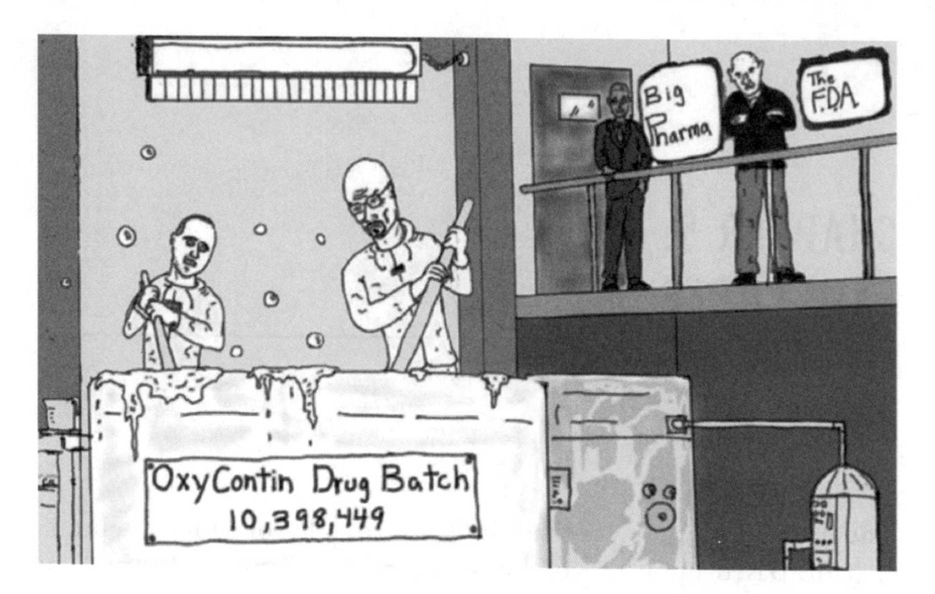


The side effects of these painkillers makes it seem like you're trading one type of pain for another. Just look at these potential side effects:

- Agitation, seizures, hallucinations.
- Lowered blood pressure and heart rate.
- Muscular rigidity and contractions.
- Nausea and vomiting.
- Non-allergic itching.
- Pupil constriction.
- Sexual dysfunction.
- Urinary retention.

Are you kidding me?

Look — you don't have to settle for a life of popping painkillers just to get through your day.

Fortunately there are natural remedies the drug companies don't want you to know about that could alleviate your pain, safely, without addiction.

## THE "WALK IT OFF" PAIN SOLUTION

"Walk it off." If you've ever hurt yourself playing sports, you've probably heard this before. It might sound insensitive, but there's evidence that shows there's some truth to it. In fact, someone telling you to walk off an injury might be the best advice you get.

The more physical exercise you do, the better you'll be at warding off pain. When you're up walking and being active, your body naturally releases endorphins. The more you walk, the more endorphins released into your system. This helps stimulate your body and produces what many people call a "runner's high."

On top of that, physical activity can help put you in a better mood. The better mood you're in, the less likely you'll notice or experience any pain. Eventually, you could train your body to endure even higher levels of pain by becoming a stronger overall person.

## "MIND OVER BODY" MENTAL TRICK TO ELIMINATING PAIN

Another phrase you might have heard if you played sports is "No pain, no gain." If you don't work hard for what you want most, you won't achieve your goals. How can you do this, however, if you're constantly facing pain every day.

That's when you need to take a "mind over body" approach. It's a natural remedy that requires you to take control over pain through willpower. Your body sends out a signal to your brain when it's in pain and centralizes it to a specific area on your body. When this happens, you need to train your brain to ignore or minimize these signals. Reducing your brain's ability to recognize these pain signals won't happen overnight. It requires practice. You might want to look into trying yoga for some of their pain management techniques.

When practicing yoga, you're training yourself to separate your mind from your body. Once you unlink the two, the pain slips away. Not only will yoga provide many health benefits for your body, it could be the secret to ridding yourself of constant pain.

## CANCEL OUT BACK PAIN WITH THESE 5 MAGNIFICENT INFLAMMATION FIGHTERS

Chronic inflammation can be debilitating to a person. Sometimes the pain is inevitable and medicine is the only way to make it manageable. But did you know there's things you can do right now that can help fight inflammation naturally? You could buy these solutions over the counter without a doctor prescription and bring temporary relief without downing a bunch of chemicals and pills. Here's 5 tips to making your life a little more pain free.

- Take advantage of fish oil and other products high in Omega 3. Omega 3 supplements assist the body with naturally reducing inflammation. It minimizes chronic inflammation and reduces pain and suffering significantly.
- Eat fermented foods, specifically carbohydrate-oriented foods. These foods help your body by supplying it with probiotics, friendly bacteria that assist with fighting the causes for inflammation. Even better, the probiotics target the gastrointestinal area, where 70% of your immune system cells are located.
- Take plant enzyme supplements. These enzymes help your body repair damaged cells that cause inflammation.
- Drink the right amount of water. Water helps your body function and can decrease the amount of inflammation from dehydrated cells.
- Take Omega-6 supplements. Foods rich in Omega-6 give your body more pain relief since most supplements high in Omega-6 contain high levels of Omega-3, another inflammation reducer. Omega-6 can also completely reduce the first stages of inflammation.

## THE SWEETEST ANTI-INFLAMMATORY ON THE MARKET

If you've been experiencing pain for a considerable amount of time, you've probably tried countless remedies to rid yourself of it. But did you know about the one pain remedy that could be sitting in your fridge right now. **Cherries**. This fruit has potent pain reducing qualities that few people are aware of. They help reduce general pain, sore muscles, and even gout.

The secret behind cherries is that they help reduce inflammation. Less inflammation in the body leads to fewer pain signals sent to the brain. You could consume this either by eating the food directly, or taking capsules which speed up pain relief.

If you're faced with constant soreness, you'll be happy to know the fruit helps relieve that pain as well. Cherries act as an amino acid and help synthesize the growth of protein in the body. The more "completed proteins", the quicker the soreness relief.

As mentioned before, cherries can help relieve pain caused by gout. It also helps with problems associated with fibromyalgia. The fruit is lower on the glycemic index, making it a great source of melatonin. This substance helps reduce pain and give you a good night sleep if you've been having trouble at night.

## THE SUPER VEGETABLE THAT CAN STOP ARTHRITIS IN ITS TRACKS

When you were a kid, you might have hated **broccoli**. But did you know that the once hated vegetable is a secret cure for arthritis pain? Some scientists have been testing the substance sulforaphane found in broccoli. They believe it could help strengthen the cartilage in your body.

If you currently suffer serious pain from arthritis, a long term diet of the green vegetable could help decrease pain. You'll notice the pain will become more mild and fade faster than before. This is because broccoli will help prevent a certain enzyme that damages cartilage from ever forming. It also helps decrease inflammation in the body.

Adding a healthy portion of broccoli to your diet could be one of the simplest steps to reducing pain and living a healthier life.

## MAKE FIBROMYALGIA DISAPPEAR OVERNIGHT

Similar to walking, when you dance, your body relieves tension as it releases endorphins. When endorphins enter your body, you might feel a "runner's high." Constant **dancing** will also reduce the amount of soreness in your body as it gets used to it. The movement will help stretch your body and make your limbs more flexible. As you begin stretching the bones, muscles, and tendons in your body, you'll begin to feel less pain.

Dancing is a great short term solution to any pain you might be feeling at the moment. If you have constant pain, adding a moderate level of dancing to your daily exercise could help immensely.

Hiring a dance teacher might be the best way to deal with long-term pain. They can teach you new ways of stretching your body and decrease pain. Certain dance moves might actually help prevent pain from even starting in the first place.

## DON'T TRUST YOUR GUT!

A common ailment amongst people all across the world, leaky gut syndrome is caused by damage to the linings of your bowel. A small hole in the intestine can cause food and other waste particles to seep through the gut and into the bloodstream. Depending on the amount of undigested food, bacteria, viruses, and toxic waste that seep into your system, you could experience various levels of pain throughout your body.

As the hole in your intestinal lining grows, the symptoms can worsen, as more and more dangerous materials escape into your system. Getting tested for **leaky gut syndrome** is the first step towards mitigating the pain. Once you're aware of the problem, inflammation and pain can be reduced almost immediately through proper treatments and/or surgery.

## WHAT CANDIDA ALBICANS CAN DO TO YOUR INSIDES

**Candida Albicans** is a harmful yeast that can find its way into your digestive track. It's could possibly cause both oral and genital infections in your body. Friendly bacteria in your system help keep your digestive system clean by feeding on and eliminating this yeast.

Certain medical treatments, such as antibiotics, chemotherapy, birth control, and cortisone lower the amount of friendly bacteria in your system, which promotes the growth of Candida Albicans. If the yeast is allowed to grow unchecked, it can travel throughout the body and damage various organs, your skin, and even your sinuses.

Checking to see if you have this harmful yeast in your body is simple. When you wake up tomorrow morning, before you eat or drink anything, spit into a cup of water. Come back and check every 10 minutes for the next hour. If you have candida albicans in your system, the water will appear to have strings dripping from the surface and have cloudy specks just below it. Your saliva will also sink to the bottom of your cup.

If your saliva doesn't sink and you can't see any string-like legs, then you most likely don't have the yeast in your system.

## DON'T LET THIS DANGEROUS SUBSTANCE BUILD UP IN YOUR BODY

If you eat a lot of fish, then you're going to want to pay extra attention. One of the biggest problems with seafood diets today is the high levels of **mercury** that makes its way into your food. Most of the time, mercury poisoning can be very difficult to cure, and most people don't know they have it until it's too late. You could avoid this danger by skipping out on seafood altogether, but there is another option available.

Mercury poisoning can be treated through mercuric chloride and chelation therapy. Though you should know that weaning your body off this poisonous substance until you're completely clean can take a long time. We're talking months to years, depending on how long you were exposed to the substance. Consult with your doctor before you decide on any form of treatment.

---

**Don't let mercury poisoning prevent you from adding fish to your diet. Adding just one meal of fish to your weekly diet could provide you with a number of health remedies. It could even prevent you from going blind!**

---

## SOME OSTEOARTHRITIS PAIN RELIEVERS

Do you suffer from arthritis? Wear and tear of your joints over the years can lead to this debilitating condition later on in life. But did you know there are natural remedies for pain caused by osteoarthritis?

Here's a number of things you can do today to help relieve pain:

- Shed Some Pounds — Losing weight is one of the simplest ways to help relieve stress on your aching joints. Did you know that for every pound you lose, you take almost 4 pounds of pressure off your knees? You might even see all your symptoms disappear if you drop 10 to 20 pounds.

- Start exercising — It might be tough at first, but coming up with an exercise routine could pay huge dividends in the long run.

- Get Over Your Fear of Needles — Acupuncture could help loosen the body and relieve stress. Some people with chronic pain found relief after trying out this ancient Chinese medical treatment.

- Glucosamine — Though there's no concrete scientific study confirming its benefits, those who take it claim it helped assist in relieving pain. Recommended dosage is 1,500mg, once a day.

- Fish or cod liver oil — A great all around natural supplement that could provide your joints the pain relief that can get you through the day.

- Chondroitin — Taking 800 to 1,200 mg a day, coupled with glucosamine, will give you the best results and could slow arthritis progression. It's a safe drug, with no side effects.

- Capsaicin cream — a topical cream that provides almost instant pain relief for muscles and joints. It's made from the same stuff that gives chili peppers its heat.

---

**These solutions might help in the long run, but if you need fast acting joint and pain relief (we're talking within 45 seconds), check out Serenity Oil Blend by The Secrets of Eden. Apply a few drops on the part of the your body that's bothering you, rub it in, and it will block the pain receptors in less than a minute.**

---

## THE REAL CAUSE OF YOUR JOINT PAIN

Sometimes that "joint pain" isn't necessarily joint pain. It could be pain coming from the tendons that within the joint. This pain could be caused by either **tendonitis** or **tendonosis**. The former is caused by inflammation of the tendon itself, while the latter is a condition where there is damage in the tendon at the cellular level. Both of these are detrimental and are often mistaken for ordinary joint pain.

Tendonitis is a rather rare condition that can take several weeks to heal. Tendonosis, on the other hand, is less severe but can persist for a much longer time. Usual recovery time for tendonosis can be several months, and even up to a year. Both problems need to be addressed and treated early on to avoid future complications.

Additionally, you should try to discover what may have caused this problem to develop in the first place. Something as simple as an old pair of shoes might create added stress on certain joints, causing damage to specific tendons. Finding the source of the problem is just as important as treating the pain it causes.

## NATURAL BONE BUILDERS YOU CAN START TAKING TODAY

Women tend to have more bone and joint problems than men. Chronic pain caused by arthritis is just as much a problem for females as they are for males. Regardless of your gender, natural bone builders can help restore bone health and maybe even alleviate nagging symptoms and other degenerative diseases. Here are a few tips that might help with any pain you might have:

- Eat foods high in calcium —This also includes milk and orange juice.You can also take supplements, but make sure they're not the only source of calcium in your diet.You need to also eat real food.

- Eat foods high in vitamin D — This nutrient promotes healthy bones. Combined with calcium, they help build stronger, more resistance bones and joints.

- Leafy greens — If it's green, it's good to eat.The green pigment in certain vegetables indicate that they're a "miracle food" that provides your body with essential nutrients. In particular, they contain high levels of calcium, vitamin K, potassium, and other vital vitamins and minerals.

Keeping your bones healthy might be difficult, but that doesn't mean it's impossible.

---

**Calcium is great, but don't rely too much on it to help build and regrow bones. Making sure you take enough magnesium is just as important in keeping your bones strong and healthy. In fact, a translation mistake in a French study led to the misconception that you need twice as much calcium as you need magnesium. The correct ratio of calcium to magnesium is 1:1.**

---

## HOW TO MAKE MIGRAINES OPTIONAL

Pain so bad you can't see. Sound is amplified to a level where you can barely function. The smallest tasks become practically impossible. Words can't accurately describe the anguish of a migraine headache. But fortunately, there's a simple natural remedy you can take that doesn't require a doctor's prescription.

It's called **Wild bergamot**, and it's actually part of the mint family. Native American groups used this herb for a number of ailments, such as cold relief and to fight bronchial infections. It's also been used to help prevent and eliminate headaches before they become debilitating. Keep it in mind the next time you're at the drug store. It could mean the difference between a splitting headache, and an calm uneventful afternoon.

---

**While we're talking about herbs, here's a list of them that lower your chances of getting diabetes: cinnamon, cloves, cilantro, coriander, cumin, fenugreek, ginseng, sage, turmeric, and lemon juice.**

---

## END MENOPAUSE MISERY

Joint and muscle aches aren't the only the types of pain you might encounter in your life. As you get older, your body's chemistry changes. And if you're a woman, you eventually have to deal with menopause. But the pain caused by the changes of hormones in your body doesn't have to be something you just grit your teeth and bear. People in societies all throughout history have dealt with the same issues, and they've discovered natural remedies that helped mitigate some of the worst symptoms.

Here is a list of herbs you can take that will help get you through some of the worst pain:

- Black Cohosh — Especially helpful against hot flashes.
- Dong Quai — Used in traditional Chinese medicine to treat gynecological conditions. Should not be used by women with fibroids or blood-clotting problems.
- Ginseng — may help with mood related symptoms and lessen sleep disturbances.

# CHAPTER 6: ALZHEIMER'S CURES

Most people don't realize how widespread Alzheimer's and dementia really is. Statistics show that in the United States, someone develops Alzheimer's disease every 69 seconds.

By 2050, this is expected to increase to a new case every 33 seconds according to the Alzheimer's Associations Disease Facts and Figures.

Around 2050, it'll be so bad, that Alzheimer's will affect one in four Americans. Thus making it more common than obesity and diabetes!

As you can imagine, most of that expected increase can be attributed to the aging baby boomer population. Even now, this disease is at epidemic proportions being that 5.4 million Americans are living with this disease.

According to a CNN report, a popular drug used to treat Alzheimer's patients in the early stages shows very little benefit — despite being approved by the FDA for moderate to severe cases. This is pretty alarming.

Fortunately Mother Nature provides solutions that are accessible to everyone to stave off this disease or even reverse it.

## THE YELLOW HERB THAT CAN PROTECT YOUR MEMORIES

Alzheimer's is a serious medical condition that many people in the U.S. suffer with. As your body slows down and ages, your brain continues to develop at a faster pace. Eventually, the brain disconnect from the body. Memory loss makes it near impossible for a person to function as they did previously.

A substance known as berberine could help mitigate some of these terrible symptoms, by providing you with lucid moments. **Berberine** is packed with a component called isoquinoline alkaloid, and it helps slow down the aging process. Isoquinoline alkaloid is made up of two antioxidants: acetylchalinesterase and butyrylcholinestaerase. They've been shown to help prevent damage to biomolecules in your body. This helps preserve memory function and lower lipids, helping with blood flow in the brain.

Adding berberine to the diet of someone suffering from Alzheimer's may help them experience more moments of lucidity.

## YOUR BODY'S NATURAL ALZHEIMER'S DEFENSE

**Creatine** is a slow-digesting protein that's been isolated and sold in over-the-counter powders for years. Originally, it was made for people looking to increase mass and bulk up. Now there's evidence showing the substance could help provide you with a memory boost.

It does more than just relieve the pain and soreness in your body. The protein also assists with cognitive function. The components in the substance work together to help the brain improve its short-term and long-term memory, especially if your body is deficient in creatine. It's still a staple for many fitness fanatics. Not only does it help improve memory function, it also helps the body grow and recover from strenuous exercise.

---

**As an added bonus, creatine fights muscle loss, increases strength, energy, and vitality.**

---

## THE JELLY THAT PROMOTES BRAIN TISSUE

**Royal jelly** is one of the most potent and complex foods you might find on the planet. The food helps with nutrient deficiencies and may also have some cognitive improvement qualities. The creamy substance is the main food source for the queen bee in a bee colony. It's naturally created by worker bees. After a queen consumes it, she can experience a 40% growth increase. Additionally, queen bees live up to 40 times longer than their worker counterparts.

The secret behind royal jelly is the acetylcholine found within it.

Increasing acetylcholine in the brain protects it from the potentially detrimental effects of Alzheimer's. Consuming royal jelly could also prevent the degenerative properties of the disease from getting worse.

## STARBUCKS' MEMORY HEALTH SECRET

If you're like most people, you have a cup of **coffee** first thing in the morning. It helps you wake up and gets you ready for the day. But did you know that cup of coffee could also be helping maintain healthy brain functions?

Studies have shown one or two cups of coffee a day help improve your brain's ability to store long-term memories. Caffeine in coffee (as well as tea) helps stimulate the parts of the brain that control memory functions.

---

**Don't stop at just boosting your memory. Add some cinnamon to your morning cup of coffee to help stabilize blood sugar for the rest of the day. This combination also reduces inflammation in the body and protects against multiple forms of cancer.**

---

## YOUR BRAIN IS SHRINKING! HERE'S HOW TO STOP IT

Every food you put into your body has a purpose. It might be something unhealthy you eat because you find it delicious. Or it might be something healthy that improves and strengthens a part of your body. You need to be aware you control everything that enters and affects your body.

For example, consuming certain **B vitamins** can boost your memory and, more importantly, slow down its natural decline. In one study, one test group received high dosages of the vitamin while another test group received a placebo. Those who received the placebo performed poorly in a number of memory and thinking tests compared to their counterparts.

For those suffering from Alzheimer's, increasing the amount of vitamin B in their daily diet could help mitigate harmful symptoms and retain lucidity.

# CHAPTER 7: MALE POTENCY CURES

Let's face it, this is not a life-threatening disease. However, erectile dysfunction is considered the most common untreated medical condition in the world. It's estimated that nearly 20 million men in the United States struggle with getting it up.

As you can imagine, most men are simply too embarrassed to discuss it, let alone visit a doctor. But — it's not something to gloss over.

ED can cause turmoil in relationships. And it may signal other medical conditions.

No doubt you can probably guess what the drug answer is for ED.

Viagra.

Just pop one of these pills an hour before sex and you're good to go. However, this drug doesn't come without costs. Besides the constant shelling out of clams to buy it, it comes with side effects which may include:

- Sudden vision loss;
- Ringing in your ears, or sudden hearing loss;
- Chest pain or heavy feeling, pain spreading to the arm or shoulder, nausea, sweating, general ill feeling;
- Irregular heartbeat;
- Swelling in your hands, ankles, or feet;
- Shortness of breath;
- Vision changes;
- Feeling light-headed, fainting; or
- Penis erection that is painful or lasts 4 hours or longer.

Less serious side effects may include:

- Warmth or redness in your face, neck, or chest;
- Stuffy nose;
- Headache;
- Memory problems;
- Upset stomach; or
- Back pain.

Did one of those side effects include "losing your soul"? Geesh… there's so many.

You've got to ask yourself the question. Do you want to spend the rest of your life popping these pills and timing your hard-on? Why do that if you can alleviate ED by fixing the root cause?

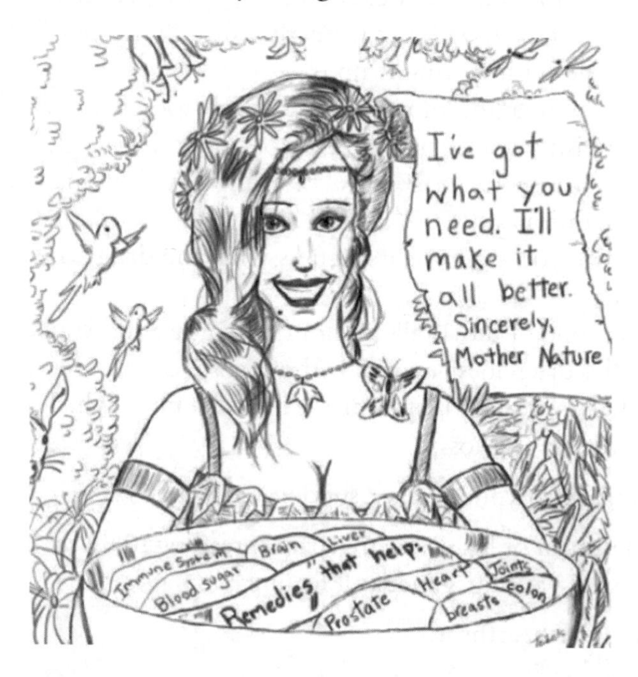


## NATURE'S VIAGRA

**Pycogenol** is a substance extracted from the bark of pine trees. It's been shown to have a wide variety of health benefits. Originally, people took it as a post-workout supplement. Trainers and other fitness enthusiasts realized the substance helped lower recovery time between workouts.

It helped prevent soreness and regulated insulin production in the body.

It was not until sometime later that scientists began looking into other possible health benefits of the extract. And they were especially intrigued when they saw it helped men suffering from erectile dysfunction. Eventually, people started calling it Earth's "natural Viagra," and many men continue to enjoy its natural benefits.

It works by stimulating the enzyme known as endothelial nitric oxide synthase. This enzyme is able to convert amino acids into nitric oxide. This helps stimulate other enzymes throughout the entire body, including sexual organs. It can even boost blood flow in men and help improve performance. Just make sure you or your partner take it an hour before you get intimate.

---

**Did you know that diabetes and atherosclerosis could actually be the cause of male impotency? These ailments cut off blood flood to the penis, making it difficult for men to achieve erections.**

---

## TWO FOR THE PRICE OF ONE!

Testosterone is one of the driving forces between masculinity and femininity in people. Men produce the hormone through the testicles, and it helps them increase their muscle mass, regulate red blood cells, grow bones, and promote their sexual drive. These are all essential when a man is intimate with his partner. The more testosterone produced in the body, the stronger the sexual desire. On the flip side, decreased levels of testosterone could lead to male intimacy problems.

There was one interesting case of a woman by the name of Alice. She went to her doctor with a number of problems. She had just recently gained 20 pounds, her had lost her sex drive, and she was afraid her husband was going to leave her. The doctor ran some tests to find out what was wrong. When the tests showed she had zero levels of one particular hormone in her system, he knew what to do.

After giving her a shot of testosterone, things quickly took a turn for the better. She lost her weight, reconnected with her husband, and found a bright new outlook on life. All thanks to a shot of testosterone.

**Testosterone therapy** can help men produce higher levels of the hormone. This gives them better performance in bed. You should know, though, this therapy should not be used by men who have had breast or prostate cancer. It would prevent the body from fighting off the disease. All other young men should take it in accordance to their doctor's advice. Testosterone levels increase a great deal via shots, patches, gels, and oral tablets. These therapy methods will help train the body to produce more testosterone without these outside factors.

---

**Before you consider testosterone therapy, here are 10 questions you should ask yourself to see if this is right for you.**

**1. Do you have a decrease in libido or sex drive?**
**2. Do you have a lack of energy?**
**3. Do you have a decrease in strength and/or endurance?**
**4. Have you lost weight?**
**5. Have you noticed a decreased "enjoyment of life"?**
**6. Are you sad and/or grumpy?**
**7. Are your erections less strong?**
**8. Have you noticed a recent deterioration in your ability to play sports?**
**9. Are you falling asleep after dinner?**
**10. Has there been a recent deterioration in your work performance?**

---

Also note that hormone replacement therapy might not be the right choice for women. One form of therapy, Pempro, could cause women to gain weight, retain fluid, increase the chance of developing blood clots, and make detecting certain cancers (like breast tumors) more difficult.

## THE HIDDEN NUTRIENT THAT CAN RESURRECT YOUR SEX DRIVE

Vitamins and minerals help your body function year round. However, sometimes it can be difficult for your body to produce enough of these vital substances to function properly. In fact, men who suffer from erectile dysfunction may have a **zinc** deficiency. So eating foods high in this nutrient could help could help correct this problem. Talk to your physician before you try anything. He or she might recommend you take over-the-counter supplements instead of altering your diet.

See your doctor if you think your zinc levels are too low. Low zinc levels and erectile dysfunction may also be symptoms of diabetes and other illnesses.

## THE THREE SECRET NUTS TO SOLID ERECTIONS

**Walnuts, pistachios, almonds** and other nuts all help decrease the symptoms associated with erectile dysfunction. Studies have even shown that they help men improve their health in up to three weeks.

The secret behind nuts is their ability to lower LDL cholesterol while promoting HDL cholesterol. Lowering the former allows the body to filter out toxins from the blood stream. This help clears out arteries, providing better blood flow and circulation throughout the body. Decreased blood flow is one of the main signs of erectile dysfunction. Improving blood could flow help lead to an increase in sexual function and mitigate other ailments.

---

**Nuts aren't the only things you can take to kickstart your sex drive. Here's 7 more potent natural stimulants you can start taking today: 1) oatmeal, 2) flaxseed, 3) chestnuts, 4) the semi-essential amino acid histidine (commonly found in chicken, saltwater fish, and soy), 5) spicy foods like garlic, onions, cinnamon, and coriander, 6) aromas like pumpkin pie, black licorice, and vanilla, and, of course, 7) horny goat weed.**

---

# CHAPTER 8: IMMUNE BOOSTERS

When penicillin was first discovered in 1928 by Alexander Fleming. It was a game-changer in how we treat infections. But for years now, rampant, over use of antibiotics has met the law of diminishing returns. Reuters reports:

> *"The more antibiotics are prescribed for coughs and flu-like illnesses, or urine infections, the more bacteria become resistant in a vicious cycle, said British researchers who analyzed 24 previous studies of antibiotic resistance."*

> *"The effect is greatest in the month immediately after treatment, but may last for up to a year, and this residual effect may be a driver for high levels of resistance in the community."*

Fortunately, more doctors are starting to limit antibiotic prescriptions.

Even still, antibiotic resistant infections now claim more lives each year than AIDS.

In a study published in the *Journal of the American Medical Association*, there were nearly 100,000 cases of invasive MRSA infections in the United States in 2005, which led to more than 18,600 deaths.

That's more than the population of Dover, New Jersey. An entire town wiped out.

When you include all resistant infections, nearly 1.7 million Americans contracted infections during hospital stays in 2007 and 100,000 people died from these diseases according to the U.S. Center of Disease Control.

This problem is costing the American health care system more than $1.87 billion a year to treat drug-resistant bacteria.

This doesn't sit well with me. There's a problem here. The so-called authorities fumbled the ball again.

We want to give you options.

## 25 QUICK TIPS

Before we get started, here's a quick shortcut. Write down these 25 super foods you can always turn to if you want to help boost your immune system. You can find them in your local grocery store, and they won't burn a hole through your wallet once you see the final bill. They are:

- Apples
- Berries
- Broccoli
- Carrots
- Citrus Fruits
- Dark Leafy Greens
- Green Food Powders
- Figs
- Dates
- Garlic
- Flaxseed
- Legumes
- Oats
- Olives
- Herbs
- Spices
- Mushrooms
- Potatoes
- Sea Vegetables

- Squash
- Tomatoes
- Soy Foods
- Nuts and Seeds
- Whole Grains
- Yogurt

## CAMPFIRE IMMUNE BOOSTERS

Boosting your immune system is the best way to prepare and strengthen your body against common ailments like the cold and flu virus. It helps increase white blood cells in the body preparing them to fight off any foreign intruders or diseases. If you imagine your body as a battlefield, boosting your immune system would be like fortifying your base defenses. And the best way to boost these defenses is by eating foods that promote and strengthen the body.

Foods like **onions**, **leeks**, and **beans**.

Onions and leeks contain flavonoid antioxidants that aid in fighting infections and bacteria by cutting down inflammation. These foods contain powerful substances like quercetin, allicin, and anthocyanins.

Beans, on the other hand, help combat cold and flu viruses. You could think of them as another "super food" due to their overall nutritional balance. Beans aid in white blood cell production, and prepares your body to be more aggressive when faced with these foreign infections.

---

**You might think getting your annual flu shot is all you have to do to keep yourself safe during flu season. But one recent study might make you think otherwise. It showed that if you vaccinate every single health care worker in a hospital, it doesn't decrease the number of flu cases at all. Why? Because unless you're one of high risk groups (children, elderly, those with respiratory problems), getting a flu shot has very little effect on whether you get sick. Just something to think about.**

---

## THE $9.99 COLD AND FLU KILLER

**Beta glucans** are a "crucial weapon" when fighting off infections and staying healthy. These nutrients come from outside bacteria sources such as yeast, grains, and shiitake mushrooms, so getting them into your system shouldn't be a problem.

This substance acts as a immunomodulator agent once you digest it. Basically, it helps promote and strengthen the immune system, getting it ready for any potential threats. They also stimulate the activity of macrophages. These are aggressive immune cells that attack pathogens that enter the body. The more beta glucans you have in your system, the more of these aggressive cells you'll have to protect you.

Beta glucans combined with antibiotics can also aid in the production of white blood cells and can beat aggressive flu viruses and diseases.

---

**Want to know what doctors do to keep themselves healthy and protected when cold season comes around? You'd be surprised at the simple steps they take.**

1. **Wash your hands**
2. **Keep all frequently used areas clean**
3. **Exercise to keep your immunity up**
4. **Take advantage of herbal medicines**

---

## THE GREAT WHITE SHARK IMMUNE INTENSIFIER

**Shark liver oil** aids in treating cancer and other diseases due to its immune boosting properties. Consuming the substance will provide you with a rich source of alkylgylcerols, a chemical that may have anticancer properties. Additionally, it will provide you with other powerful nutrients that can combat other diseases.

Recent studies also show that shark liver oil could inhibit the growth of tumors in blood vessels. The oil lined the walls of these blood vessels, preventing excess tumor forming proteins from forming. Certain studies have also shown that when used in combination with chemotherapy, patients had a better chance of seeing tumors shrink or disappear completely.

## THE COLD AND FLU CURE FOUND IN THE PRODUCE DEPARTMENT

People have been enhancing their food with spices throughout history. You might be surprised, however, to find out many of these spices have positive health benefits. In fact, there's one spice used in countless dishes all over the world that could help boost your immune system and protect you against some forms of cancer.

**Garlic:** In a way, it's an elixir in herbal medicine. The cloves help fight against the common cold and keep other infectious diseases at bay. A single clove of garlic has 5 mg of calcium, 100 sulfuric compounds and 12 mg of potassium. Combined, these ingredients are a powerful natural remedy and can clear out bacteria and infections from the body. Raw garlic was even used to help prevent gangrene in both World Wars, showing just how powerful it is as an ingredient.

---

**Garlic is just one spice you can take to slow down the aging process and add years to your life. Think about incorporating the following spices into your diet to keep your body young and active: turmeric, basil, thyme, cloves, oregano, sage, rosemary, ginger, cinnamon, chili pepper, cayenne, and capsaicin.**

---

## HOW HONEY CAN PROTECT YOU FROM THE FLU

**Manuka honey** isn't like the regular honey you buy in the grocery store. The honey is created by bees in New Zealand who feed off the nectar of the manuka tree. The honey contains a substance called methylgloxal, a compound that assists with antibacterial activity.

When you eat this honey, your body produces something called cytokines. This substance helps the body organize and prepare the immune system, improving your body's natural response. The honey also assists with healing chronic wounds. Recent studies have shown it kills about 85% of bacteria that develops a biofilm. Biofilm is a substance that allows bacteria and other microorganisms to stick together, making chronic wounds more prevalent.

Consuming this honey will also boost the immune system, getting it ready to deal with any pathogens that enter the body. A tablespoon a day can help the body significantly, especially when mixed with cinnamon and water.

## THE EMPHYSEMA FLU-BUSTER

Amino acids and antioxidants are essential in the daily bodily functions. **N'acetylcystein** (NAC) is a super substance that can help protect you against colds and flus. Studies have shown that amino acids and antioxidants reduce and loosen mucus of people who suffer from chronic bronchitis. NAC can help naturally break down the buildup of fluid in your body and relieve congestion.

Additionally, NAC protects the liver from damage caused by acetaminophen by creating a protective lining around it. It also increases your resistance against particular nasty strands of flu (such as the H1N1 virus, commonly known as "swine flu") and boosts your overall immune system. It promotes the production of glutathione, another powerful and important antioxidant in the body.

---

**What happens if you come down with the flu, you take your temperature, and you discover you're running a high fever? If it's over 104 degrees, you should go see a doctor. But for anything below that, the best thing you could do is... nothing. Fevers usually run their course in a day or two.**

---

## BOOST YOUR IMMUNE SYSTEM WITH THIS LITTLE KNOWN BERRY

**Elderberry** is a handy option for people with autoimmune disorder or people who have weak immune systems and are susceptible to colds and flus. When you consume elderberry, the substance assists the body with the production of cytokinesis. Cytokines are proteins that help regulate and stabilize various systems in the body and help your immune system fend off diseases and infections.

When administered in effective dosages or with the drug, Sambucol, elderberries create a powerful autoimmune response that has improved the lives and health of AIDS and cancer patients. It's best to use over the counter pills or syrup when ingesting the substance.

Studies are still ongoing and clinical trials are in order. Regardless, current tests show it's an effective immune booster.

---

**Check out these other food options to help strengthen your metabolism and aid in digestive recovery: yogurt, kefir, kombucha tea, kimchi, and sauerkraut.**

---

## DON'T OVERLOAD ON FIBER!

High levels of fiber in your diet help regulate bowel flow and improve your intestinal health. The better your bowel movements, the healthier you are, in general. Now there's even claims of weight loss benefits associated with it. However, care should be made not to ingest too much of the substance.

One reason why fiber is so popular for people trying to lose weight is because it makes you feel more full. Fiber fills you up and prevents you from overeating. If you consume more than a normal amount, you could cause health problems like cramping. This occurs when the body can't properly break down and synthesize foods. Just like the old saying goes, too much of anything is bad for you. And that certainly applies to fiber. In fact, significantly high levels of fiber in your system may stop the digestive process completely.

## THE SUN DETOX

When you hear people talking about ultraviolet light, they're normally talking about its negative effects. But did you know that in moderate dosages, this light can actually have some positive health benefits.

If you're looking to detox your body from harmful toxins, UV light might be the best way to go. For example, **photoluminescence**, a form of UV therapy, can help eliminate botulism poison from your body within 24 to 72 hours. Studies have also shown that no other type of therapy is as effective as ultraviolet therapy. Consult with your physician to see if this option is available and whether it can improve your health.

# CHAPTER 9: MISCELLANEOUS CURES AND THINGS TO WATCH OUT FOR

## 3 WAYS TO PREVENT SURGICAL MISTAKES

Doctors might have dedicated a large portion of their lives learning their trade, but that doesn't mean they're perfect. And while you should trust your doctor's doing his or her best to make you better, there are things you can do to make sure mistakes aren't accidentally made. Here are a couple of surgical mistakes to watch out for to prevent a potential malpractice suit.

- Require Automated Surgery Scheduling — If you've ever tried to read a doctor's handwriting, you'll know why this is important. Scheduling a surgery through a computer ensures that all parties can understand what needs to be done, and can avoid confusion and chance once you're on the surgical table.

- Help Your Doctor Out — If you're having surgery on your right knee, make sure you mark it yourself. No one else cares about your body as much as you do. So many sure you do everything you can to eliminate risk before you go under.

- Don't Rush Pre-Op —Your doctor is working for you, make sure he goes over everything before the operation.

---

**Before you go under the knife, you should know there are some surgeries you should avoid if possible.**

---

**1. Stents for Stable Angina — if you're having a heart attack, a stent can be a lifesaver. But in cases of stable angina, it's no better at preventing a heart attack or prolonging life than regular exercise and taking statins.**

**2. Complex Spinal Fusion for Stenosis — some doctors believe this surgery will prevent back pain caused by stenosis, but there's no general consensus on the best way to treat that type of pain.**

**3. Hysterectomy for Uterine Fibroids — this type of surgery increases a woman's chances of incontinence by the age of 60.**

**4. Knee Arthroscopy for Osteoarthritis — this surgery involves placing a tiny camera in the knee and then using small instruments to repair torn or aging cartilage. Regardless, it's no more successful than non-invasive remedies.**

## STOP WASHING YOUR HANDS!

Washing your hands might not be as beneficial as your mother told you. **Triclosan**, an antibacterial compound found in most hand sanitizers, has a number of detrimental effects you don't normally read about. It might "disinfect and kill 99.9% of all germs," but at what cost?

The substance can cause chronic skin irritation if used for a prolonged period of time. Additionally, some bacteria might develop resistance against the compound, giving you a false sense of security. It could even disrupt the natural function of your body's endocrine system.

## HOW TO STAY ON YOUR TOES AND PREVENT BALANCE ISSUES

Back in 2010, the government reported that 2.3 million Americans suffered from some sort of non-fatal fall. Over 600,000 of those people had to spend some time in the hospital because of their injuries. While they survived, these mishaps can be expensive. On top of that, the constant fear of losing your balance can take its toll on your daily life.

A study released by Harvard Medical School might have found the culprit behind many of these falls. The researchers believe certain types of medication might be affecting a person's balance, making them more likely to suffer from an accident.

The following medicines might be affecting your balance:

- antidepressants
- anti-anxiety drugs
- antihistamines prescribed to relieve allergy symptoms
- blood pressure and other heart medications
- pain relievers, both prescription and nonprescription
- sleep aids (over-the-counter and prescription forms)

Also note that a combination of these medicines might have negatives effects. Talk to your doctor if you think your balance issues might be caused by one of the medications you're currently on.

## WHY YOU NEED TO KNOW WHAT ANTICHOLINERGIC DRUGS ARE?

There's a type of drugs that might be sitting in your medicine cabinet right now that could increase the risk of cognitive impairment. In other words, it could affect your ability to think. A number of drugs such as anti-depressants, bladder medication, heart medication, painkillers, and antihistamines contain a substance known as an anticholinergic.

People with long-term use of this substance are more likely to develop dementia than those who are not exposed to it. Here's a sample of some common drugs that contain the anticholinergic agent:

- Symmetrel
- Elavil Asendin
- Sal-Tropine
- Cogentin
- Dimetapp, Lodrane
- Tegretol
- Histex, Carihist
- Chlor-Trimeton, Chlophen
- Thorazine
- Tavist
- Anafranil

- Clozaril
- Flexeril
- Enablex
- Norpramin
- Bentyl
- Dramine
- Benadryl
- Senequan, Zonalon
- Urispas
- Atarax, Vistaril
- Anaspaz, Cystospaz, Levsin

If you can live without these drugs, then it's probably best to avoid taking them.

## BEST "BEFORE BED" FOODS

Sometimes the best meal of the day is the one you have right before you go to sleep. A lot of people will tell you that eating right before you call it a night is bad for you. But they're wrong. In fact, certain foods will actually help with digestion while you're asleep. Check out this list of healthy late night snack foods.

- White meat protein — If you have any chicken leftover in the fridge, don't feel guilty about warming up a plate of it. Your body digests this high protein food slowly. This allows your stomach to work while you're resting, so you won't wake up feeling starved.

- Cottage cheese — Another great protein source. Eat it plain and try to avoid adding any unneeded sugar.

- Low-carb protein shakes — If you have any creatine available, make yourself a smoothie and throw in some of the potent powder. This will sit well in your stomach and allow your body to process fats. It will also keep your metabolism running high throughout the night.

- Green vegetables — Nothing is better than getting a couple of servings of green right before bed. They're excellent sources of protein and they're not too high in calories.

- BONUS: Want to make sure you get a good night sleep, even with your late night snack? Turn off the TV and make sure it stays off. Watching TV stimulates the brain and makes it more difficult to relax and fall asleep.

---

**Throughout this report, we've told you about a number of foods commonly thought to be unhealthy. Feel free to add them to your list of "before bed" foods. They include: chocolate, coconut milk, grass-fed beef and butter, and whole eggs with the yolk.**

---

## THE ANTI-DIET FOODS

A diet is a great way to get healthy and shed excess pounds. But before you start stocking up on so-called "diet" foods, you need to be careful about what you buy. Just because a company says their food is good for your diet doesn't actually mean they're healthy. It's important to know what makes up a healthy diet, as opposed to just buying "diet" products. Here's a list of some foods to watch out for.

- Breakfast cereal — they're loaded with sugar and refined carbs. In other words, they're not good for you. These types of cereals have been known to cause insulin blood spikes, causing you to crash later in the day, most likely right as you're walking into the office.

- Agave nectar — many people will rave about the health benefits of the nectar, but take that advice with a grain of salt. Agave nectar, on average, is about 70–90% fructose. Compare that to sugar, which is only 50% fructose. A diet that contains high levels of fructose could cause your body to develop a resistance to insulin.

- Whole-Wheat Bread — The term whole-wheat bread is just

a marketing gimmick made to give the impression that their bread is healthier than its competitors. Whole-wheat bread is healthier than refined wheat, but that really doesn't mean much. If you want a healthy bread option, look for anything made with whole-grains, like Ezekial Bread. You can even get Ezekial flourless tortillas if the recipe calls for it.

- Granola — Unless it's homemade, stay away from the granola you find in stores. The stuff you find in the supermarket has added sugars and oils, things that ruin any healthy diet.

Also, watch out for foods like low-fat yogurt, commercial salad dressing (even the low-fat kind), store-bought fruit juice, diet soda, organic processed food, trail mix, and gluten-free cakes and cookies. Here's a simple rule of thumb. If your great-grandmother wouldn't recognize it as food, don't eat it.

---

**Losing weight is great... but there's an even better reason to cut back on sugar in your diet. It could be increasing your chance of developing certain cancers. In the words of Dr. William Campbell Douglass II, M.D., the man who's been called the "conscience of modern medicine,": Sugar is practically Miracle-Gro for many types of tumors. Additionally, cutting out sugary sodas could reduce your risk of developing diabetes by up to 83%.High fructose corn syrup, what soda companies in the U.S. use as a substitute for sugar, is the one carbohydrate you should avoid at all costs.**

---